Bioresonance:
a new view of medicine

Scientific principles and
practical experience

Dr. med. Jürgen Hennecke

For Simone

Bioresonance: a new view of medicine

Scientific principles and practical experience

Dr. med. Jürgen Hennecke

© 2012 Jürgen Hennecke
Trans-shipment, production and publishing: Books on Demand GmbH, Norderstedt
ISBN 978-3-8448-2375-2

Bibliographical information of the German National Library
The German National Library has listed this publication in the German National Bibliography; detailed bibliographical data can be obtained on the internet at http://dnb.d-nb.de.

The scientific observations made here are presented by the writer to the best of his knowledge. The case studies reported here are descriptions of the author's own cases or a general portrayal of other therapists' cases from publications.
Neither the publisher nor the author accept responsibility for the prognosis or treatment of specific medical cases. This lies in the hands of the attending doctor or therapist.

Contents

Broadening our horizons	7
How it all began...	9
From an idea to an approach for therapy	13
Medicine becomes physical	17
Outstanding medical technology	29
How the bioresonance method functions	41
On the trail of hidden causes of disease	53
Swift help	61
The new widespread disease	65
From hay fever to asthma	69
Our largest organ – the skin	75
Problems in the digestive tract	79
Pathogenic influences at the workplace	83
Allergological detective work	87
Own cells under attack	93
Latent adverse effects from pathogens	99
Hidden poison	107
The sensitive nervous system	113
Pain warning signs	119
Degenerated cell growth	125
When enjoyment becomes an addiction	129
Bioresonance babies and the change of life	133
Problems in the mouth area	137
Our four-legged and feathered friends	145
What evidence is available?	155
Frequently asked questions	179
Concluding remarks	187
Glossary	189

Broadening our horizons

First contact with bioresonance

My life was to change on 11 November 1988. I came into contact for the first time with a method of therapy which, at the time, was completely new to me but which was to profoundly influence my future professional and private life.

Up to that point I had studied medicine in the conventional way, completed the training to become a specialist in general medicine and had set up my own medical practice two years previously. I had taken an interest in alternative medicine at an early stage, started training in acupuncture, explored various other 'natural' methods and gained the additional designation 'naturopathic practice'. Ever since my school days I had been interested in the natural sciences and the structure of our universe. Astronomy was my hobby and the theory of relativity and quantum physics had fascinated me. It was initially a purely theoretical interest since these scientific discoveries did not appear to have any direct relevance for our everyday life. After all, you can get by in everyday life very well with the classical laws of physics and chemistry.

What led me to this meeting in a hotel in Aachen back in November 1988 was not just the friendly persuasion, on the telephone, of an employee of the bioresonance firm but my increasing frustration with the limitations of the treatment offered by conventional medicine. I was, and still am, fully committed to operating as a practitioner of conventional medicine within the state insurance scheme and am very taken with scientific advances within modern medicine. However, this does not mean that you have to restrict yourself to this approach and cannot risk broadening your horizons. I won't deny a certain amount of curiosity either.

So now there it was in front of me, this amazing bioresonance device. After a few introductory words the company's representative carried out some muscle tests, acupuncture point measurements and trial treatments on me. Although I had not completely understood it all, I was definitely interested and I experienced that indefinable gut feeling which said: "You've got to have this!" After a brief period of consideration I bought it and several weeks later was sitting with my wife in the

Broadening our horizons

introductory seminar by Lake Starnberg, where a new world was opened up to me. I learnt here how, through the bioresonance device, the fascinating laws of quantum physics can be applied to everyday practice in a manner which appears almost magical. Here we met physicists, doctors and therapists who not only introduced us to the theory but also reported astonishing success with therapy.

It was admittedly at first not easy to incorporate the new approach into our daily practice. We had a lot to learn and built up our own experience. The big breakthrough came in the early 90s. New practical discoveries brought unbelievable results, especially in the treatment of allergies. News of the bioresonance method quickly spread by word of mouth and soon patients were waiting weeks for an appointment to have their allergies 'zapped'. We needed more therapy devices, took on additional staff and the demand still hasn't tailed off. Bioresonance is such a successful method of treating patients that I cannot now imagine it not being part of my practice.

> Frustration, scientific interest and curiosity led the author to discover more about bioresonance, a method which was new to him but which has since become well established in his practice.

How it all began...

Historical review

In the 1950s reports and ideas of an unusual method of treatment reached European shores: **acupuncture**, an important component of Traditional Chinese Medicine, with a history dating back over 4000 years. The first pioneers in this field were eyed critically by conventional medicine. However, they proved not only to be enthusiastic disciples of this method, they developed new and creative ideas based upon it. This theory revolved around strange acupuncture points apparently linked with one another by a kind of 'energy transport channel', the undetectable acupuncture meridians. Clever 'researchers' soon discovered that skin resistance at these acupuncture points differed from skin resistance of neighbouring tissue. And what's more: conclusions could be drawn from the changes and fluctuations in potential at the point regarding the energy content of the meridians and thus the state of health of the associated tissue or organ. Values which were too high were evidence of a pathological process just as much as readings which were too low.

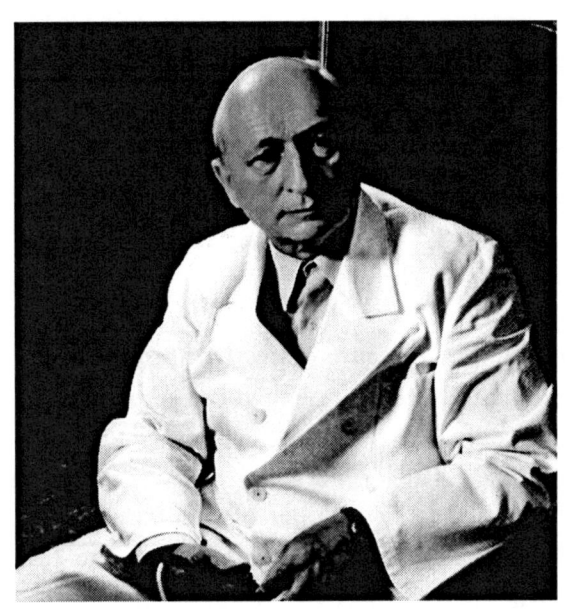

Fig. 1: Dr Reinhold Voll developed the electro-acupuncture method named after him (EAV).

The German doctor **Dr Reinhold Voll** deserves the credit for having researched and systematised this application. He not only discovered important energetic connections between meridian points, tissues, organs and teeth, he also detected additional points and new meridians outside the classic Chinese pathways. This method is still taught as **Voll's electroacupuncture (EAV)** and used with positive results.

As with many other scientific discoveries, an element of chance played a part in the further development of this EAV method. Dr Voll tested a patient and detected a pathological reading at a point on the liver meridian. When he repeated the test a few minutes later, the reading was suddenly in the normal range. Dr Voll was astonished and at first presumed that the initial pathological reading had been incorrect. Then he noticed that the patient was holding a homeopathic remedy in her hand. Dr Voll asked her to put down the remedy and the reading promptly returned to the pathological range. Touching the remedy again resulted in an immediate improvement in the reading. But that was not all: it emerged that the information from the remedy could be transmitted not just by direct physical contact but also by a cable connected to the measuring device.

Voll's medication test which was subsequently to become famous had been discovered.

It was now possible to develop a new system for diagnosing and treating patients: over 300 acupuncture points were measured on the bodies of sick patients and a homeopathic remedy (individual or complex), capable of bringing these points into the normal range, was tested out for all the pathological points. This medication (sometimes consisting of 20-30 substances) was then administered to the patient, generally in the form of injections. A very laborious yet, as it emerged later, also very effective method of treatment, free from adverse side-effects.

The German doctor **Dr Franz Morell** was a pupil of Dr Voll and an enthusiastic exponent of electroacupuncture. Together with his son-in-law **Erich Rasche**, an electrical engineer, he developed a medication test transmitter with which the information from the medication could be transferred to a test person standing further away without using cables. In so doing he proved that the effect of homeopathic remedies must be attributed to ultrafine electromagnetic oscillations.

The field strength must be so weak that it could not be measured directly by any conventional device. The effects on the living organism could however be deduced directly from the changes in the test readings at the acupuncture points.

Dr Morell went one step further. He pondered the large number of medicines to be used and asked himself: if information from medicines significantly alters the test readings, then very similar information must also be present in the body. If this information is picked up straight from the body and modulated in a particular way, then a similar phenomenon should occur to that produced in medicine testing.

How it all began...

Consequently, together with Rasche, Dr Morell built a device designed to pick up information from the body and return it following modulation. The device was called the MORA device after the first two letters of its developers' names. An electrically conductive electrode was placed on the skin of the affected part of the body and the information fed into the Mora device through a cable. This information was 'inverted' inside the device by means of 'phase shifting' and fed back to the body via a different electrode. Astonishingly this led in most cases to an improvement in the patient's state of health or even a full recovery. Once again a new method of treating patients had emerged.

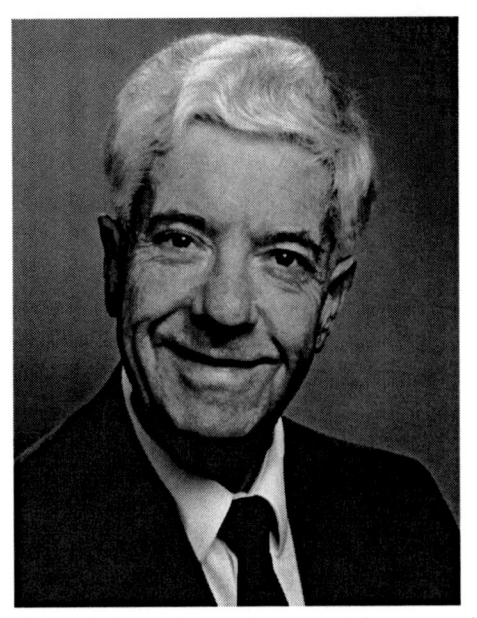

Fig. 2: Dr Franz Morell discovered therapy with information from the body's and substances' natural oscillations.

Thanks to technical advances in subsequent years, especially with the advent of the computer age, the Mora device was developed further and its operation improved. A new name was coined for this method of therapy: **bioresonance (or also bioinformation)**. The names are intended to indicate what it's about: **reson**ance phenomena in **bio**logical systems through the transmission of **information**. Scientific working hypotheses describing this phenomenon weren't to come till much later.

Bioresonance devices are now manufactured and marketed by a number of different firms. The experiences described in this book were obtained using the **Bicom bioresonance device**. The word Bicom is a coined term and one which is protected under trade mark law.

> Dr Voll developed electroacupuncture in the 1960s and discovered the non-material medication test. Based on these ideas, Dr Morell, together with the electrical engineer Rasche, developed a device which treated patients with information from electromagnetic oscillations. It was from this that the bioresonance method of therapy developed.

From an idea to an approach for therapy

Following on from Dr Morell's inspired idea, numerous doctors and non-medical practitioners have advanced this method of testing and treating patients through their own research and by accumulating experience, by trialling and testing and a great deal of deliberation and even more intuition. Bioresonance is an empirical method which is categorised as experienced-based medicine. Since this method initially lacked a convincing scientific explanation and a theoretical framework, bioresonance was largely developed purely as a result of the practical experience of its users. Mention should be made here of the non-medical practitioner Gerda Otten, who introduced the idea of using the body's natural substances and proposed applying propolis as a substance with an antibiotic effect.

Various special electrodes were developed as early as the 1980s such as rigid and flexible electrodes, magnetic electrodes, dental and spectacle-type electrodes. A major advance at this time was also the elaboration of indication-based therapy programs. A therapy program describes the manner in which information fed into the device is modulated by the device in order to be returned to the patient as a therapeutic impulse. It is defined by programming a particular type of therapy, a frequency, an oscillation amplitude and the therapy time.

The contribution of the Austrian non-medical practitioner Sissi Karz should be recognised here. Through tireless experiments, tests and no little intuition she has developed over 400 therapy programs which, based on years of positive experience, can still be retrieved from the Bicom bioresonance device. Recently over 150 programs from the low deep frequency range have been added. In addition Frau Karz has proposed a therapy system which focuses on the use of the body's natural frequency patterns, also deploying the patient's own fluids (blood, urine, stool, etc.). The aim is to improve the body's ability to regulate itself by consistently using the body's own 'pharmacy' (according to Morell's theories).

In spring 1987 Dr. Morell made a landmark announcement during a seminar. If the information from allergens such as pollen or foods affecting the patient was applied to the patient after appropriate modulation by the device, virtually all the electroacupuncture

From an idea to an approach for therapy

test readings moved into the normal range. This marked the beginning of a new era for allergy therapy.

Dr Peter Schumacher, a paediatrician from Innsbruck, conducted extensive research for a number of years on this basis and in 1991 published a sensational study on biophysical allergy therapy. He presented an approach whereby allergy could be treated with considerable success through a combination of strict avoidance of allergens and consistent bioresonance inverse oscillation. He observed that chronic allergies to cows' milk and wheat, often combined with Candida fungal infestation, are partially responsible for many diseases which prove hard to treat. He demonstrated in an effectiveness study which he conducted himself that a success rate of up to 90% could be achieved in children with neurodermatitis, bronchial asthma and hay fever.

In 1991 I applied an idea of the kinesiologist Jimmy Scott[1] to bioresonance therapy and was also able to achieve highly effective allergy therapy, in some cases even without allergen avoidance, by 'flooding' certain acupuncture meridians. Working together with my wife Simone, new therapy programs and systematic approaches to therapy were developed.

A further development of Dr P. Schumacher's approach was presented a short while later by Dr Th. Klein and Dr P. Schweitzer. By improving the transfer of information from the allergen into the device through 2 cables and from the device to the patient through spherical electrodes and by increasing the amplification of the therapy amplitude, it was also possible to achieve more effective allergy therapy. A series of additional proven allergy therapy programs was subsequently proposed by various users.

The German doctor Dr G.L. Rummel presented his own alternative approach in the mid 1990s. His basic idea is that the structure of the constituents of cows' milk and wheat resembles the structure of all other relevant allergens. If you treat patients sufficiently often with a combination of the counter oscillation of cows' milk and wheat, combined with biophysical Candida therapy, virtually all allergy-related diseases can be treated.

---

[1] Jimmy Scott, Kathleen Goss: Allergie und der Weg, sich in wenigen Minuten davon zu befreien {Allergy and how to overcome it in just a few minutes}, Verlag für angewandte Kinesiologie, Freiburg.

From an idea to an approach for therapy

In persistent cases the patient is then also treated with virus nosodes[2]. The considerable success achieved with over 20,000 recorded cases treated speaks for itself. This is an approach which is easy to carry out yet which sometimes requires considerable time.

The non-medical practitioners Martin Keymer and Dieter Kramer developed therapy ampoules for systematically testing and treating stresses which cause illness in patients. In this procedure information with a positive effect on the meridian and organ areas is applied to the patient to stabilise energy levels. Inverting the negative oscillations of toxins and pathogens during the same treatment session relieves the body and restores the cells' ability to regulate. The non-medical practitioner A. Baklayan sees infestation with parasites as one of the main causes of chronic disease and devised an approach with appropriate test ampoules.

I hope the many researchers and users who I have not mentioned or named personally will forgive me. The wide variety of approaches shows that bioresonance therapy is not an inflexible and dogmatic method but that, once the basic training has been completed, there are many different possibilities for therapy. The method is developing dynamically and this is an ongoing process.

Further significant advances have been related to the technical development of the Bicom device: the infrared transmitter for wireless transfer of information contained in ampoules, programs for analogue potentiation, micromagnetic field therapy integrated in the device, use of low deep frequencies and an additional second therapy channel for stabilising the patient during therapy.

> Based on the empirical experience of numerous creative practitioners and following technical advances, the bioresonance method has developed into an effective method of diagnosing and treating patients. Various therapy systems now exist which are continuously being developed further.

---

[2] Devitalised microbial cultures of pathogens, potentiated according to homeopathic principles, and of pathogenically changed organic material and of toxic substances.

Medicine becomes physical

The biophysical mode of action

The triumphant progress of the natural sciences began at the end of the 18th century. Numerous discoveries resulting from observations, reproducible experiments and mathematically definable laws of nature flooded every domain of physics, chemistry and biology. The scientific laws of nature calculate and confirm the things which we perceive with our senses or whose effects we can feel directly. These are the laws of nature which are taught at school and university and which we know from our everyday lives. These are the laws of nature which mankind has used to build huge skyscrapers, to fly to the moon or to develop modern computer technology.

Enthusiasm for these developments and their applicability to daily life has led many to take the view that everything – absolutely everything – in this world can be explained by these laws. Much can be calculated and explained. However, there are effects and processes which strangely do not fit into this scientific world view. "I only believe what I can see or measure or demonstrate" is the motto of a whole generation of contemporaries, especially of scientists, researchers and doctors. For the time being paranormal phenomena and alternative medicine have no place in this 'materialistic' world view and, consequently, are quickly dismissed as superstition and quackery – or else ignored completely.

For around the last one hundred years branches of science have developed alongside traditional natural science which appear to provide a totally different view of our universe. These include Einstein's general and special theory of relativity which showed that even space and time are relative terms. Quantum physics proved that elementary particles can be described as both waves and particles.

String theory tries to unite the two partially conflicting views and describes all elementary particles and rays as tiny vibrating threads (strings). These are just a few examples of a new perspective on the physical world. Matter is therefore just a small part of a universal energy. There are blurred relationships and probability structures, multiple dimensions and the relative passage of time. The laws of classical physics and chemistry are no longer applicable in the microcosmos of elementary particles.

Medicine becomes physical

In many areas oscillatory information and resonance phenomena appear to direct the world. Countless theories, many of them contradictory, show that there is a lot we still do not know and there is a huge need for further research.

The formula to explain the world has not yet been found. But one thing is clear. "There are more things between heaven and earth, than are dreamed of in our book learning" (Goethe). Why do these pioneering findings occupy such a niche existence in our lives? Why do so few people know anything about the fringe sciences? Why is this not taught at school and university? One reason may be that the connections and the associated mathematical formulae are either still too complicated so that even scientifically trained individuals have difficulty fully understanding them or reconstructing the thought processes. Or they simply do not want to admit that some pieces are still missing from the scientific puzzle. This makes it easier not to accept certain phenomena.

There are now several excellent books on the fringe sciences, however. Another reason may perhaps be that we have the impression that these could be quite interesting topics for a philosophical discussion over a glass of wine by the fire but they have little relevance to our everyday lives. Furthermore, social learning teaches us to condemn challenges which shatter our 'accepted' world view in a certain way, as being undesirable or beyond the acceptable norm. Even some acknowledged pioneering scientists sometimes feign inexplicable ignorance. Perhaps they are also afraid of losing their reputation.

If we deal with alternative medicine, the discoveries of quantum physics, for example, acquire relevant importance. The key to acceptable theories of the ways in which homeopathy, acupuncture and bioresonance work may lie in this field. Let us now summarise the most important factors for us to comprehend:
Our universe consists of energy in the form of matter and interactive quanta and information. The ratio of matter to interactive quanta is around one to one billion. This means that matter, as a kind of 'frozen energy', represents just a billionth part of our universe. All types of energy behave in physical terms both as particles and as oscillating fields. The term 'information' has not yet been clearly defined from a physical viewpoint. Some scientists regard information as a special form of energy. Others do not actually see energy in information, yet assume that all processes between elementary particles are controlled by information.

Medicine becomes physical

Modern computer technology shows us how it is possible to store an incredible amount of information in a tiny space. Would we have believed 20 years ago that the works of an entire library would fit on a stick measuring just 1 cm² and could be retrieved with incredible speed? And this performance can be improved even more with future 'quantum computers'. But nature has long been able to achieve what we can do today through technical advances. Individual elementary particles (such as a photon) can store an unbelievable 10^{127} (that's one with 127 noughts!) bits of information. Life on earth would be inconceivable if information were not transferred in a perfect and sophisticated process.

One of the key substances for the emergence of life on our planet is **water**. It covers 70% of the earth's surface and the first life forms developed in the primordial oceans. Even we humans are made up of over 70% water. Many branches of science are now looking into the unusual properties of water. The behaviour of liquid water differs in every respect from that of other liquids. This includes maximum density dependent on temperature and viscosity determined by pressure.

Water is the only substance that is lighter in its solid state than when liquid. This is why icebergs can float and lakes freeze over from the surface downwards. This is how fish can survive the winter in streams and lakes. Many researchers believe the reason for these anomalies lies in the physical properties of **hydrogen bridge-type bonds**.

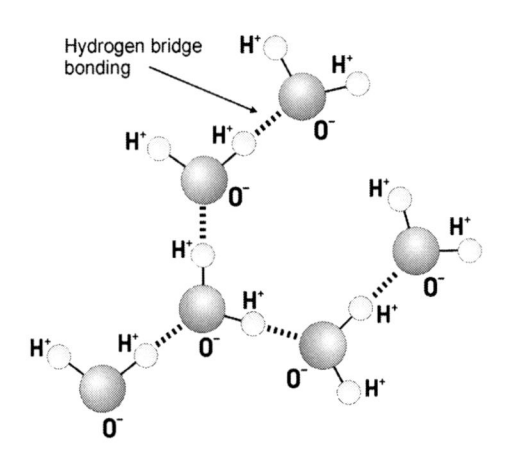

Fig. 3: Hydrogen bridge bonding: the electrical attraction between positively charged hydrogen atoms and negatively charged oxygen atoms leads to the development of water structures of varying stability.

As we all know, the water molecule H_2O consists of one oxygen atom and two hydrogen atoms. The oxygen atom is negatively and the hydrogen atoms positively charged. The bilateral forces not only hold the individual water molecule together but form bonds of varying strength with the neighbouring molecules. This results in the formation of molecular chains which can form various spatial structures. A tetramer of four water molecules can form as many as four different shapes (chain, ring, star and lasso) and tetrahedrons. These extended molecule complexes are called **clusters** and are now the subject of scientific research. The numerous spatial structures of smaller clusters of up to twelve molecules can be calculated mathematically. Larger clusters form icosahedral networks of 280 and more water molecules and can be examined using laser spectroscopy.

A variety of cluster structures can be detected in water in its liquid state, dependent on pressure, temperature and external influences. When foreign atoms or molecules occur in the liquid solution, new cluster structures immediately form around these 'intruders'. These newly formed clusters may be very robust and able to be detected even if the atom responsible is no longer present in the liquid. Each cluster structure has its own specific frequency spectrum. It is possible to imagine what vast quantities of information can be stored in the three-dimensional, multi-molecular cluster structures. And one can also imagine that cluster structures can be built up or destroyed through resonance phenomena (homeopathy and bioresonance) with specific frequencies.

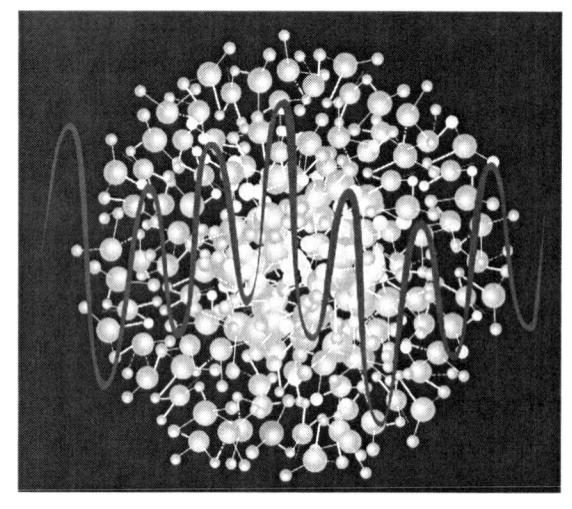

Fig. 4: Cluster model: spatially structured collections of water molecules can store information.

In 1988 Jacques Benveniste together with ten other scientists published a paper on 'water's memory' in the scientific journal Nature. He was accused of being esoteric by representatives of 'official' science and lost his laboratory and funding. The biochemist Prof. Madeleine Ennis wanted to disprove the effect of homeopathy and diluted substances in water until no molecule of the substance could be detected or measured. Contrary to expectation the specific biological effect of the original substance was still present in 'pure' water. The results of this experiment were confirmed in double blind trials conducted in four other laboratories in France and Italy. It was possible to delete this memory by heating these solutions to over 70 degrees Celsius and by low frequency alternating magnetic fields. Does this destroy the specific cluster structures?

Medicine becomes physical

Benveniste went one step further. He wound a coil around the glass vessel containing the homeopathised solution and fed the information it contained to a glass vessel with a second coil by means of an amplifier for electromagnetic oscillations. The previously 'uninformed' solution now displayed the same biological properties as the substance in the first beaker. The transfer of information was interrupted by covering and screening the vessels. Benveniste concluded from this that water's memory and its transfer was in some way related to electromagnetic oscillation.

Experiments by Anderson, Reid and Bill[3] demonstrated similar phenomena. NaCl (salt) dissolved in water usually forms cubic crystals. If large molecules such as proteins (e.g. serum albumin) are added to this solution, the crystal formation is modified to a widely ramified, dendritic (fernleaf-like) crystalline form. This technique is used in gynaecology with cervical smears to determine the point of ovulation. Astonishingly this information for different crystal formation was transferred from one salt solution to another via a platinum gold wire (without an electric current!). Dendritic salt crystals now also formed in the 'informed' solution without the material presence of proteins.

Prof. C. W. Smith[4] conducted similar experiments with patients in England. These were people with severe food allergies who reacted with violent symptoms to the slightest amount of their allergen. The allergens were diluted homeopathically and administered to the patients. It emerged that certain dilution stages (potentiations) triggered allergic reactions while other dilutions improved these reactions or caused them to disappear. This effect was even triggered with dilutions beyond 10^{23} (see Loschmidt number), i.e. if the solution no longer contained any molecules of the original substance – further proof of the 'memory' of water. Prof. Smith repeated these experiments using a frequency

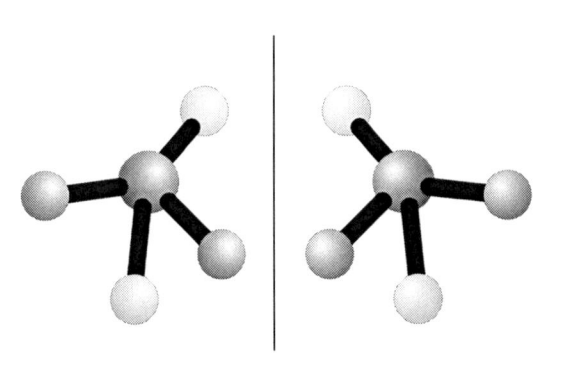

Fig. 5: Chirality: chemically identical molecules differ in the spatial arrangement of their atoms (e.g. mirror image).

---

[3] Vicinal, long range and extremely long range effects on growth of sodium chloride crystals from aqueous solutions containing protein; Applied Physics Communications 4, (2-3), 217-239, 1984; The Ability of an Electric Current to Carry Information for Crystal Growth Pattern; Journal of Biological Physics 15, 33-35, 1987.

[4] C. W. Smith: Elektromagnetfeld- und Bioresonanzeffekte im lebenden Organismus [Electromagnetic field and bioresonance effects in living organisms], Erfahrungsheilkunde, p. 237, 4, 1993.

generator. It emerged that certain (likely) frequencies of the allergen trigger allergic reactions while other frequency ranges can 'heal' these. Were electromagnetic oscillations or frequency patterns obviously triggering biological reactions in the body here too? How significant are these oscillations for the functioning of our cells?

But it isn't just water which is able to absorb, store and then transmit information in the form of electromagnetic oscillation patterns. All organic biomolecules such as amino acids, sugar and nucleotides have this potential. 'Handedness' (cf. chirality) obviously plays a major part here. Almost all spatially asymmetrical molecules can occur in two mirror images thereby creating a virtually identical match. We know this from yoghurts with 'right-spin' and 'left-spin' lactic acid. Chemically the two lactic acids are completely the same, only their spatial structure is opposite (like a right and left glove). In living organisms one of two spin directions is preferred and only this can be utilised in metabolism. These asymmetrical molecules not only have a considerable storage capacity, they also form large helical giant molecules.

A special role is attached to the spiral giant **DNA** molecule (deoxyribonucleic acid) whose base sequence encodes our entire genetic potential. The spatial structure of DNA evidently acts like a mini antenna through which the cell can communicate with neighbouring cells and also with distant tissue.

Prof. Fritz-Albert Popp deserves the credit for having detected electromagnetic oscillation patterns, emitted by cells, in the form of light particles or light quanta (photons). He called these **biophotons**. According to his investigations they are essential for cell metabolism to proceed in a regulated manner. More than 10,000 biochemical reactions take place every second in each cell. And these are not chaotic but ordered in a strictly hierarchical system. Chemical or enzyme reactions would be much too slow for this purpose. According to Prof. Popp the only possibility is that a superordinate electromagnetic oscillating field regulates all metabolic processes via biophotons.

How do the body's small cells find the information intended for them out of the billions of pieces of oscillatory information surrounding them? The mystery is resonance, a concept familiar to you from music and acoustics, for example. It is the same principle by which a television selects the right broadcast that you want from the range of hundreds of stations/programmes received in parallel. Or a mobile phone that finds the right person from millions of communications across the globe. All this can only work if the frequency patterns of the transmitter and receiver resonate exactly with one another or have been coordinated accordingly. And nature has been capable of this for a long time.

Cells communicate with one another and with their environment by means of ultraweak signals. Some researchers assume that one single photon is sufficient for this. If the cell's receiver system resonates with the incoming information, this can trigger a whole cascade of biochemical metabolic processes. This is the purest form of **bioresonance**.

Many pioneering experiments have now been published supporting the assumption that micro organisms and cell groups communicate without matter.

For those readers interested in the science, some pioneering experiments with astonishing results are touched upon below. If you find this too boring or complicated, you can skip the following paragraphs.

A Japanese research team experimented with the bacterial strain Bacillus carpo-philus Kasumi. This only survived on culture media containing salt if carbon was also added. The culture medium was divided and only one half of the bacterial strain received the vital carbon. To the astonishment of the scientists the other half without the carbon also survived, even when the bacterial colonies were separated from each other by a glass or plastic wall. The authors came to the conclusion that the survival of the bacteria without carbon was only possible through the transfer of vital information by physical means from one bacterial colony to the other.[5]

In another experiment human white blood cells were incited by the substance phorbol 12-myristate 13-acetate to release reactive oxygen species (ROS) abruptly. It was also possible to provoke this reaction in an impressive manner by transferring the non-material information from the substance to the solution with the white blood cells using an audio amplifier.[6]

---

[5] Michio Matsuhashi et al.: Studies on Carbon Material Requirements for Bacterial Proliferation and Spore Germination under Stress Conditions: A New Mechanism Involving Transmission of Physical Signals; Journal of Bacteriology, p. 688-693, 1995.

[6] Y. Thomas et al.: Activation of human neutrophils by electronically transmitted phorbol-myristate acetate; Medical Hypotheses, 54(1), p. 33-39, 2000.

In addition to DNA molecules, cell membranes obviously also play a major part in the electromagnetic transfer of information in the living organism. The concentration of glucose in the blood first produces oscillations of the transmembrane potential in the cell membranes of the pancreas (islets of Langerhans). These then act on cell metabolism, causing the release of insulin.[7]

Back in 1979 Nelson and Henkart demonstrated that mesenchymal cells respond to external stimuli with a dramatic increase in cell membrane potential. The oscillations of the membrane potential are transferable from cell to cell. Within the cell they cause a rise in the concentration of potassium ions. These in turn regulate the function and structure of the cytoskeleton, which generates the shape of a cell. The shape of the cell is closely connected to the metabolic processes in the cell itself.[8] This study therefore shows that the oscillatory information of the cell membranes is responsible for regulating the entire biochemistry of a cell.

Experiments were conducted in the Institute of Physics at the University of Marburg which demonstrate the crucial significance of the natural oscillations of all cellular membrane systems. ATP synthase is a membrane protein (enzyme) which converts ADP (adenosine diphosphate) into the energy storage molecule ATP (adenosine triphosphate). When protons enter through the cell wall, parts of the ATP synthase are set rotating. Since this molecule projects partly into the cytoplasm (cell fluid), this is also set flowing. As a result they form a biological oscillatory system and, through currents, the flow of protons creates an electromagnetic field. Here we have an example of how living organisms can create bioelectric fields.

The significance of these mechanisms is clear from experiments on embryogenesis. In the absence of the abovementioned rotation systems, malformations occur such as the placement of organs within the organism on a purely random basis.[9]

These examples of basic experiments by renowned scientists and institutes from around

---

[7] E.K. Matthews and M. D. L. O'Connor: Dynamic Oscillations in the Membrane Potential of Pancreatic Islet Cells; Journal of Experimental Biology, 1979. Vol. 81, 75-91.

[8] P. G. Nelson and M. P. Henkart: Oscillatory Membrane Potential Changes in Cells of Mesenchymal Origin: The Role of an Intracellular Calcium Regulating System; Journal of Experimental Biology, 1979. Vol. 81, 49-61.

[9] P. Lenz, Department of Physics: Biologische Motoren [Biological motors], Physik Journal, 2004. no. 6, 41-46.

the world are included to show that investigation of electromagnetic control frequencies in the organism is now quite mainstream and the evidence is growing that electromagnetic oscillatory information plays an important part in cell metabolism and in cell communication. Other scientists point out that, in addition to electromagnetic oscillations, other oscillatory information which has not yet been investigated in detail could play an additional role.

These research results are the basis for explanatory models of physical oscillation therapies such as homeopathy and bioresonance. If it is possible to influence the superordinate 'oscillation field of life' by means of appropriate impulses, we can also modify the biochemical processes in the body by the same method.

A comparison with computer technology which is familiar to everybody will clarify these mechanisms for the less scientifically minded:

Imagine the body were a computer. The programs for all the biochemical reactions for metabolism and the hormone and immune system are stored on the hard drive (memory). Connecting to the internet (outside world) results in repeated infection with computer viruses, i.e. parasitic programs, which can disrupt or paralyse the proper functioning of the hard disk. A good anti-virus program with regular updates (immunesystem) safeguards the computer against most attackers without any problem. Yet sometimes the security system fails and malfunctions are inevitable. The best solution would now be a suitable 'counter program' which rectifies the malfunction and deletes or eliminates the computer virus program. In the worst case scenario the whole system crashes. In that case the only solution is for the (computer) clinic to replace the hardware in the same way as a drug treatment or surgical intervention.

If we take the example of a hayfever sufferer, stored in his body's cells is the allergy program: "birch pollen causes the impulse to sneeze." If we succeed in deleting this disruptive program with an appropriate counter program (cf. positive computer antivirus), then the impulse to sneeze no longer occurs the next time the patient comes into contact with birch pollen. A model which is certainly considerably simplified, yet easy to understand: the body computer's hardware represents the molecules of the cells of the body while the software represents the superordinate electromagnetic oscillatory field with its pre-loaded programs. Germs, toxins, malfunctions of the metabolism or of

Medicine becomes physical

the immune system cause disruptive programs which lead to physical (in the example, apparently ridiculous) symptoms. Eliminating the disruptive program with a suitable electromagnetic impulse which resonates 'positively' can restore the body's natural regulation and help the body to recover.

Now we just need to know how to successfully create these electromagnetic healing impulses technically.

> Over the last hundred years revolutionary fundamental research has amended the previous world view of classical physics and chemistry. Oscillatory information now plays an important part in all material and also biological systems and even appears to fulfil a superordinate control function. Explanatory models for forms of alternative medicine such as homeopathy and bioresonance can be derived from this.

Outstanding medical technology

The mode of operation of the bioresonance device

The mode of action has been clear since Dr Morell first had his inspiration: electromagnetic information is picked up from the patient or a substance using electrodes, 'modulated' in the bioresonance device and then 'applied' to the patient or an information carrier. The first Mora device was relatively straightforward in its construction: incoming information was modulated by phase shifting, amplified and applied via one of the eight available frequency ranges (low frequency 'low pass' or high frequency 'high pass'). Technical advances on the one hand and the increasing need for differentiated treatment strategies for patients with multiple problems on the other hand led to devices becoming ever more technically sophisticated. The most important technical details will be explained here through the example of the Bicom bioresonance device.

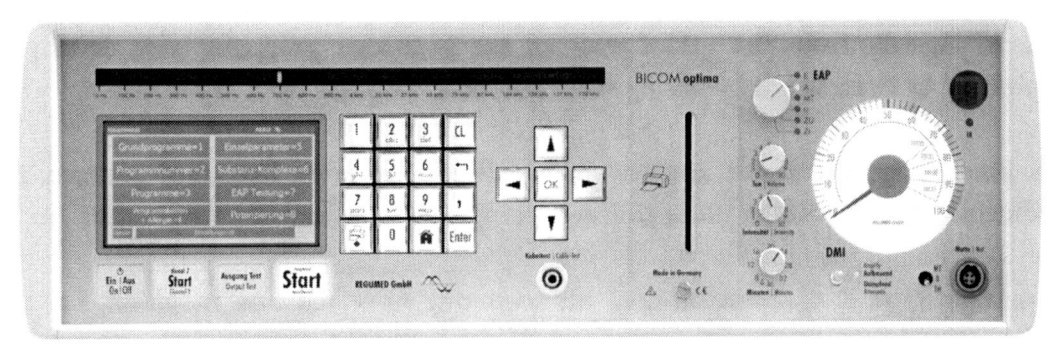

Fig. 6: A modern bioresonance therapy device – Bicom Optima.

Scientific 'experts' who examined the Bicom device with their measuring apparatus were agreed: the device is a 'black box'. Nothing goes in and nothing comes out. Just like the attitude: "Something I can't measure doesn't exist!" This approach is reminiscent of the fisherman who fishes in the lake with his 10 cm mesh fishing net and doesn't catch anything. His verdict, "there are no fish in this lake!" because he was unable to catch the thousands of fish smaller than 10 cm, appears ludicrous to us. Consequently certain expert opinions on this issue seem rather naïve and, above all, unscientific. In fact the volume of the electromagnetic oscillatory information with which the device operates is so low that it is generally lost in the ambient noise and cannot (yet) be measured with the instruments customarily available today. Despite its low volume the body can identify it, due to its specific frequency pattern, and respond. Our body is the most sensitive measuring instrument we know.

Another misjudgement of the bioresonance method can be seen in the following question which is often raised: "How can the device identify what I have and then treat me correctly?" Of course the device cannot identify anything, it is just as stupid as any computer. It is only capable of modulating incoming information as instructed by the therapist and passing it on. Compare it with a mirror. A mirror reflects all the incoming light particles (photons) without having 'analysed' them beforehand. The reflected image can be modified (modulated) depending on the colouring, shape and curvature of the mirror. Here are a few details for those readers interested in the technical aspects.

A specific **therapy program** predetermines how the frequency patterns coming into the device (device 'input') are modulated. Each therapy program is defined by certain parameters: a therapy type, a 'bandpass' (selected frequency band), amplification (amplitude) and therapy time. The action of a program in the body cannot always be deduced logically from the parameters. All the preloaded programs were developed empirically, in other words by testing them out, observing and from experience.

The **therapy type** describes the way in which the incoming frequency patterns are modulated: with or without phase shifting, all together or selected by a separator?

In **therapy type A (All unchanged)** the incoming wave remains 'in phase', i.e. the basic pattern of the oscillation is retained. If the incoming and outgoing waves were laid on top of each other, we would basically see the same wave pattern. This essentially supports the body's natural or the substance's natural oscillation pattern. With this therapy type the energy levels of physiological organ function can be improved or information from medication with a positive influence (homeopathic remedies, organotherapeutics, phytotherapeutic remedies, etc.) can be applied. With pathological information therapy type A can also be used for 'provocation', e.g. in patients with blocked reactions or to detect residual conditions caused by pathogens or toxins.

In **therapy type Ai (All inverted)** a phase shift around 180 degrees is generated technically. The incoming frequency patterns are **inverted**, i.e. the outgoing oscillations

Outstanding medical technology

are upside down in mirror image. Minus becomes plus and plus becomes minus. If the incoming and outgoing waves are superimposed one on the other, the frequency pattern is inverted exactly. At first it was believed the pathological frequencies in the body were deleted by interference from these oscillations and that this explained how bioresonance operated. This theory would not hold scientifically however. Now we tend to assume that the way the information is stored in the water clusters is altered. Therapy type Ai is used, amongst other things, to treat disrupted organ function, to treat allergies and intolerance and to eliminate toxin and pathogens.

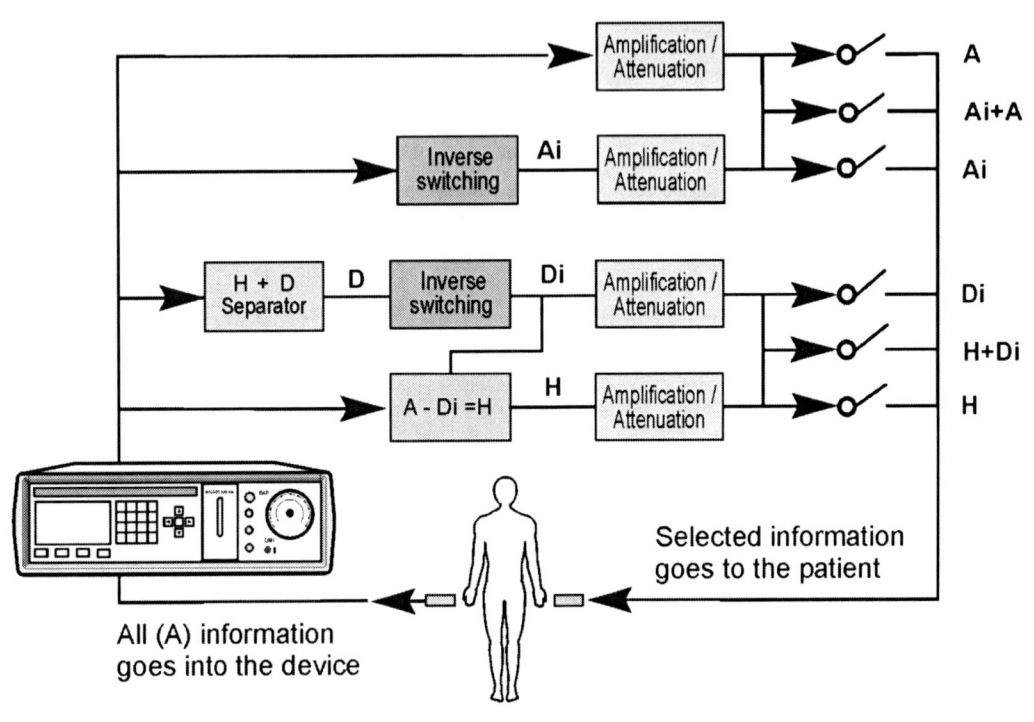

Therapy types:

A   = All frequency patterns not inverted
Ai   = All frequency patterns inverted
Ai+A = Both elements (Ai+A) alternately
D   = Pathological elements
Di   = Only pathological elements inverted
H   = Only physiological elements
H+Di = Physiological elements and
        inverted pathological elements

Fig. 7: Therapy types of the Bicom bioresonance device.

Outstanding medical technology

The Bicom device also contains a **separator,** a biological filter system for frequency patterns. This filter can separate two basic oscillation patterns from one another: physiological and pathological frequency patterns. The healthy or physiological frequency patterns which tend to be regular and ordered used to be called 'harmonious', hence the designation H. Note also: **H** as in 'health'. In contrast the rather irregular, chaotic, unhealthy or pathological frequency patterns were called 'disharmonious' and designated with the letter **D**. Think of the word 'disease'.

It is possible to apply **therapy type H** on its own. The patient receives only physiological oscillations, with the pathological ones being filtered out. Based on this type there are restorative programs for patients who are exhausted or suffering from severe stress.

In **therapy type Di (D inverted)** only the pathological frequency patterns are applied. Indications include the treatment of interference fields, acute conditions and infections with pathogens.

Therapy type H + Di combines these two functions. The physiological oscillations are unchanged, possibly amplified, while the pathological oscillations are applied inverted. This is a wonderful harmonising of energy levels which is used with a wide range of indication-related programs.

Therapy type Ai − A is a special feature. Here the A function is squeezed in for a few seconds at regular intervals during Ai therapy. The aim is to deliver energetic provocation and this has proved beneficial with regulatory blocks and patients affected by residual toxins or pathogens.

The **frequency range** is an important parameter for bioresonance therapy. It describes a specific 'wave function'. If you throw a stone into the water, small waves form on the surface of the water extending outwards in rings. The distance between the peaks of the small waves is the **wavelength**. If you now count the waves which hit the shore each second you have the **frequency**. This is measured in **Hertz**; one wave per second is one Hertz, ten waves per second is 10 Hertz etc.

Frequency is in inverse proportion to wavelength. Long waves have a low frequency, oscillations with a short wavelength have high frequencies. This also applies to sound

Outstanding medical technology

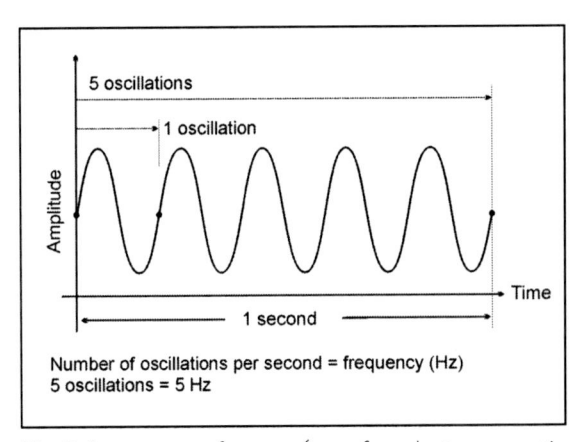

Fig. 8: Parameters of a wave (e.g. of an electromagnetic oscillation).

waves and electromagnetic oscillations. The oscillation spectrum of electromagnetic waves consists of frequencies from below 1 Hz to 10^{23} Hz[10]. Out of this spectrum our eyes can only detect the visible light of 384 kHz (red) and 789 kHz (violet). Specific measuring instruments are required for lower wavelengths like infrared and radio waves and higher wavelengths from ultraviolet to X-rays. Our earth's atmosphere also acts like a radiation filter and only allows two wavelength ranges through to us. These ranges are named **Adey window** after the person who discovered them.

If we assume that electromagnetic oscillations (biophotons) play a superordinate part for biological metabolic processes, the corresponding frequency ranges must also be considered in therapy. The frequency ranges between 10 and 150,000 Hertz (150 kHz) which are relevant for therapy have been used in the Bicom device for years. Their use has led to astonishingly successful treatment. Due to technical advances with the latest electronics in 2009 the bandpass (a narrow frequency range which lets through information) was extended to the range from 1 to 10 Hertz (Bicom Optima).

The significance of the low deep frequencies will be explained by way of some examples. Our brain operates predominantly in the low frequency range. Beta waves (14-30 Hz), alpha waves (7.5-14 Hz), theta waves (3-7 Hz) and gamma waves (0.5-3 Hz) can be differentiated by EEG (electroencephalogram). Very low frequency ranges occur frequently during meditation and sleep. Low frequencies are also easily transmitted in the earth's atmosphere. The lower layers of the atmosphere act like a cavity resonator here. An important frequency range for life on earth is the **Schumann waves** from 7.5 to 7.8 Hz named after their discoverer. The first astronauts in space had health problems because they lacked these important frequency ranges. Consequently modern space stations always contain a Schumann frequency generator.

---

[10] The wavelength above the UV range is normally referred to as radiation and wavelengths below infrared beams as waves.

Outstanding medical technology

Now back to the Bicom device. The use of low frequencies resulted in marked progress in the use of bioresonance. The Bicom Optima has around 150 new programs in the low deep frequency range. In some therapies the entire frequency range of the information entering the device is modulated simultaneously and fed back again as a therapy signal. This takes place through the device setting: **All frequencies** or **No bandpass**.

It often makes sense, however, not to treat the entire frequency range simultaneously but one after another. For this a narrow bandpass runs through the entire frequency range from 10 Hz (in the Bicom Optima 1 Hz) to 150 kHz from bottom to top and back again. This has a crucial benefit. Prof. Smith and his colleagues discovered that the body resonates with appropriate therapy signals within a fraction of a second while unsuitable frequencies require significantly longer time to take effect. In this **continuous band pass** or **frequency sweep** the optimal therapy signals are already filtered out, as it were, by briefly touching the effective frequency ranges. This setting is used in basic therapies, amongst other things, and when testing and treating with specific test ampoules.

Treatment with a very narrow frequency range (**manual** setting) is often more effective for specific diseases. Not only organs, tissues and meridians, but also pathogens and disease-induced changes caused by acute or chronic inflammation have their highly specific frequency range in which the signals are transmitted. The relevant bandpass can be selected by testing or from experience so that the affected tissue can respond to this impulse in the best possible way by resonating

A **bandpass** is a technical means of allowing through only a small frequency range from the entire frequency spectrum. A centre frequency is set in the device and the **fixed narrow bandpass** lets only this frequency pass with a tolerance of 4.5% above and below. If a larger frequency range around the centre frequency is required, then increased tolerance of around 20% can be achieved with the setting **wobbling narrow bandpass.**

The **amplification** parameter describes the amplitude of the oscillation, in other words the height of the peak of the wave. In a radio this would equate to the volume control. If the volume is too low we don't hear anything and if it is too high it is not exactly pleasant for our eardrums. Just as there is an optimum range for the volume of music, so the cells respond best to a certain signal strength of electromagnetic oscillations. Impulses which are too weak have no effect while those which are too strong block metabolic activity. In the Bicom device amplification 1 means that the amplitude of the outgoing oscillation matches that of the incoming information exactly. It is technically possible to reduce the amplification to 0.025 (on H to 0.1) and increase the amplitude to 64 (H to 12.5). Most disease-specific programs are programmed to a **constant amplification**.

Elimination of toxins, pathogens, intolerance and allergies often requires treatment at several amplification stages. Consequently it is also possible to **increase and reduce the amplification stage** in the Bicom device. Here the amplification is automatically switched up or down to double or half the amplitude for a certain period (e.g. a minute).

The **amplification sweep** enables the various amplifications to be applied continuously rather than in stages. Any intermediate stages required are included in this setting. In **increasing amplification sweep** the amplification slowly rises to the selected upper limit (max. 64), drops immediately to the starting point, rises again, etc. This gives a 'sawtooth-like' amplification pattern. In **decreasing amplification sweep** (only available in the Bicom Optima) the amplification is reduced from high to low. In the H+Di setting there is a reciprocal amplification sweep. Here the therapy type Di increases while the H information simultaneously decreases in reverse or reciprocally. In **increasing and decreasing amplification sweep** the sequence of amplification changes always rises and falls alternately. These variations have proved effective especially with allergy therapy.

Therapy signals can be applied **continuously** or in the form of **interval therapy**. In the latter small breaks are built in at regular intervals so that the cells can briefly recover and can possibly process the subsequent signals better.

The **therapy time** for the preloaded programs is set for an average patient. If necessary it can be reduced or extended. Half the therapy time is often sufficient for children.

Three different therapy programs can be entered in the Bicom device (six in the Bicom Optima) and these are then applied automatically one after the other. There are recommended therapy program combinations for the most frequent indications for humans and animals. In the Bicom Optima these combinations are already preset as **program series** making practical implementation easier.

Outstanding medical technology

Proven therapy combinations includes **smoking cessation treatment, weight loss program** and several **applications for wellbeing, health spa treatments** and **fitness**.

Analogue potentiation of substances is an independent treatment strategy. 'Potentiation' is a term from classical homeopathy. It refers to the step by step dilution and succussion of a substance, generally in an alcohol water solution. In this process the material content is continually reduced yet, from an energetic viewpoint, the substance becomes an extremely effective medication. The water cluster compounds which were described earlier are presumed to be the mode of action. The energetic structure of a potentiation can be imitated by the Bicom device with special program parameters. The mineral solution now applied has similar properties to the corresponding potentiation stage. It is obviously not a genuine potentiation yet has a very similar effect and is therefore called 'analogue potentiation'. Analogue potentiation stages from D3 to D1000 are possible. The body's natural secretions (blood, urine, pus, stool, etc.), medicines, toxins and pathogens are used as original substances.

Special **electrodes** which conduct electricity are used to transfer information from the patient into the Bicom device (input). If possible, they should make direct contact with the skin or mucous membranes. It is worth repeating at this point that there is **no current** flowing in the cables between the electrodes and the device. There are flat metal electrodes for hands and feet, cylindrical and spherical electrodes, pointed electrodes for teeth and acupuncture points. Flexible electrodes of differing sizes are used for the trunk and joints while a pinhole glasses electrode is employed for eyes and nose. These electrodes can all also be used at the device output, in other words to transfer information from the device to the patient.

Usually the **modulation mat** is used for this however. It is a special output electrode with a micromagnetic field. This magnetic field has a very low field strength (less than the earth's magnetic field) and is therefore safe to use on patients with pacemakers. It has considerable depth of penetration however and a very potent biological effect on all tissues and organs. The mildly stimulating action on the circulation is desirable but contraindicated in patients with acute haemorrhaging. The modulation mat has two functions which are independent of one another and can consequently be applied separately if necessary. The main task is to convert the therapy information modulated in the output to the micromagnetic field to then be applied to the patient (**BMF – Bicom magnetic frequency pattern**).

Outstanding medical technology

The second function of the modulation mat, independent of the first, is **dynamic micro-magnetic field impulse therapy (DMI)**. Here an external magnetic field pattern, independent of the patient, is applied, to 'prepare' the terrain energetically, as it were. Through the **strengthening** setting, exhausted patients are given a frequency pattern which alters from low frequencies and amplifications to high frequencies and amplifications as well as information from the energising precious stones ruby and fire opal. Patients with excess energy can be helped with the **attenuating** setting. Here the frequency patterns of high frequencies and amplifications are shifted down and information from the precious stones onyx and black tourmaline is applied.

All the information running through the modulation mat can be simultaneously transferred to a metal chip via a chip storage device. This is stuck on the patient's body to prolong the treatment over the days when no therapy is administered. Mineral solutions and skin oils can also store therapy information and are readily used to supplement therapy.

Another important element is the **cup electrodes.** For therapy programs related to organs or disease the body's natural secretions are added to the **input cup**. Blood, urine, saliva, sputum, earwax, hair, nails as well as wound swabs, pus, surgical material, extracted teeth, etc. are used depending on the indication. Information from these secretions assists the therapeutic effect considerably. Also added to the input cup however are substances required for therapy, either supportive medication, organ or meridian ampoules or pathological information such as ampoules of toxins, pathogens and allergens.

It is also possible to connect the input of the Bicom device to a PC or laptop and to deliver the physiological or pathological substances to the device in **frequency patterns** that have been **saved digitally** (e.g. via Multisoft software). This digital information is of the same quality as that of the test ampoules. In this way a large number of substances can be tested very quickly and neatly at the touch of a button or mouse click. The relevant conditions can also be treated directly through the computer via a pilot program. A wonderful solution for computer freaks. The **Multisoft software program** holds over 6000 test substances stored digitally.

The new Bicom Optima also has a **second input** with a special **honeycomb** as input cup. Via this channel and using an A program stabilising frequency patterns can be applied at **the same time**, such as the information from organ and meridian ampoules,

Outstanding medical technology

medication, probiotics, colours and precious stones, flower essences, etc. This not only saves a considerable amount of time, it intensifies the therapy and reduces the risk of hypertensive reactions.

The output cup has a similar function to the chip storage device. Mineral solutions, oils, ointments, neutral globules, medication, etc. can be added here for the patient to use on days when no therapy is being administered to prolong and intensify the treatment. Just to recap: liquids can store information through the cluster structure of water.

BICOM Multisoft	

Cause-related basic test
    Outline testing of adverse influences
    Physical exertion
    Focal toxicoses
    Immunology
    Toxicology
    Allergy
    Orthomolecular substances
    Miasms
Indication-related basic test
    Outline testing of organ areas
    Pathogens by specialism
        Dermatology
        Gastroenterology
        Haematology/immunology
        ENT
        Cardiology/pneumology
        Infections
        Nephrology
        Neurology
        Ophthalmology
        Oncology
        Orthopaedics
        Paediatrics
        Metabolism
        Urology/gynaecology
	BICOM setting
	Therapy
	    Therapy programs
	    Individual therapy
	    Potentiation programs
	EAP testing
	    Carry out test
	    Analyse list
	    Analyse graphics
	    Differences left/right
	    Differences before/after
	    Analyse quadrants
	Combined test technique
	    5 feedback circuits - human
	    5 feedback circuits - horses
	    5 feedback circuits - dogs
	    5 feedback circuits - cats
	    Allergic conditions
	    Inhalational allergens
	    Parasites/ environmental contamination
	    E numbers
	    Inoculations/ metals
	    Bacteria
	    Viruses/ fungi
	Patients' master data

Fig. 9: BICOM Multisoft.

Outstanding medical technology

The therapy program parameters resulting from empirical research, such as therapy type, frequency and amplification and their biological action, are explained through the example of the Bicom bioresonance device. Specially adapted electrodes are used to transfer information.

How the bioresonance method functions

Therapeutic and practical use

A Bicom bioresonance session generally starts with basic therapy. At this first stage of therapy it is not yet about treating a specific tissue, organ or disorder. It is a non-specific program which sensitises the body's cells for further therapy and prepares the 'sound board'. The aim is to bring a little more order into the chaos in this first step. The basic therapies are therefore programmed to amplification sweep and continuous bandpass. This means that all the frequency ranges between 10 Hz and 150 kHz are treated. The low deep frequencies from 1 Hz to 25 Hz can also be treated with the Bicom Optima. An electroacupuncture examination on a series of patients showed that significant improvements were achieved in the values measured at a number of acupuncture points simply as a result of basic therapy. This would suggest an improvement in the flow of energy within the body.

In the case of **acute disorders, indication-based follow-up therapy** is usually used after basic therapy. This is selected on the basis of proven recommendations or after testing by the person treating. There are preloaded programs for acute infections, inflammation, joint and back pain, etc.

In the case of **chronic disorders**, it makes sense to follow a therapy system. There are various recommendations for this based on the experiences and methods of long-standing users and which are taught at the relevant seminars. Over the course of several therapy sessions the various energetic stresses affecting the body are treated step by step. This includes removing therapy blocks (radiation exposure, scar interference fields, spinal blocks), improving the functioning of organs and meridians, detoxifying and eliminating toxins, treating allergies and intolerance, eliminating environmental toxins and pathogens and removing interference fields and foci.

One of the most important therapy blocks is **chronic radiation exposure**. This topic is still widely disputed in the press and scientific circles. However there are numerous reports which describe the negative effects of electromagnetic fields and warn of their impact on health. Many therapists operating with naturopathy have long known that

How the bioresonance method functions

this radiation exposure is not only involved in triggering or aggravating some diseases but that regulatory methods of therapy do not 'work' so well on these patients. There are excellent Bicom programs which remove the effects of radiation exposure thereby making subsequent follow-up therapy more effective. Yet this obviously does not remove the cause of the problem. A geobiologist should be called in if the patient is severely impeded. In over 90% of cases the place where the patient sleeps is the main problem.

In the active phase of life during the day the body is in a state of sympathetic activity and fortunately is able to compensate fairly well for the radiation now constantly surrounding us everywhere. During the night-time resting phase we switch to parasympathetic tone, lie for eight hours or more in the same place and our cells are supposed to recover from the stress of the day. Yet how can they do this when they continue to be 'irradiated' in this phase?

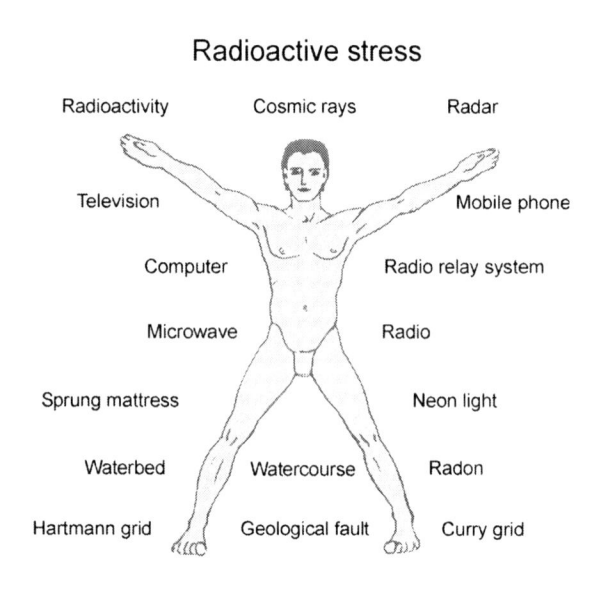

Fig. 10: Radiation exposure can damage health and impede effective therapy.

There are two main groups of radiation: electronic smog and geopathy. 'Electronic smog' covers a large group of electrical, magnetic and electromagnetic static or pulsed alternating fields which have now flooded all areas of our lives and which we can no longer avoid. This includes computers, TVs, radios, mobile phones and their radio masts, cordless telephones, W-LAN and much more. Geopathy covers radiation that has existed from time immemorial from watercourses, geological faults, intersections of grid networks (Hartmann, Curry, Benker), radon, cosmic radiation, etc. Both types of radiation may have a damaging effect on health in the long term with individual resilience varying considerably. While some patients feel no direct adverse effect, others complain after just a short time of disturbed sleep, nightmares, pain in the joints and back in the morning, etc.

How the bioresonance method functions

The job of the geobiologist is to track down the cause in situ with rod and measuring instruments, to change the position of the bed and take appropriate steps to remove the interference. Oscillation neutralisation is an interesting principle. It has been known since ancient times that the oscillation of some semi-precious stones (rose quartz, tourmaline, malachite, etc.) can protect the organism from the influence of 'bad radiation'. Following this basic principle, mixtures of minerals, metals and precious stones packaged in wooden balls or little bags are now available. While these interference suppressers are not able to neutralise any radiation present, they can however protect the organism so that the radiation which still exists no longer has a negative impact. The **biosafe** is a wooden ball prepared according to this principle and filled with a specific mixture of precious stones which is used by many therapists to stabilise the atmospheric energy at the place where bioresonance is to operate.

Scar interference fields are also important therapy blocks. Scars consist of fibrous filler which spans defects in tissue and organs. Any scar following surgery, an accident or severe inflammation can basically act as an interference field. When tissue is injured, small nerves and blood vessels are damaged. The flow of energy in acupuncture meridians is also interrupted. This may result in local impaired functioning such as motor disturbance, pain and sensory disturbance. Remote disturbances have also been observed. Consequently a scar on the appendix may cause constipation, back pain and knee problems.

Removal of scar interference has played a large part in neural therapy for years. Scars are injected with procaine or some other local anaesthetic. The 'Huneke phenomenon' named after its discoverer, whereby symptoms improve immediately after an interference field is injected, has become famous. The change in membrane potential of the cell membrane caused by the neural therapeutic is assumed to be the mechanism causing this effect.

A comparable effect can be achieved with bioresonance therapy. Scar interference is suppressed permanently following repeated use. Some patients report a marked improvement in their symptoms merely from removal of scar interference. One patient complained of severe pain and restricted movement in the left shoulder after surgery for breast cancer. Following bioresonance programs to suppress scar interference, the pain had virtually disappeared and she could move the shoulder freely. Another patient's

How the bioresonance method functions

constipation improved dramatically once the scar on the appendix was suppressed. Bioresonance is particularly suitable for patients who are afraid of injections and for children. Treatment of lower abdominal scars so common in women and which often cause problems is as neat and pain-free as treatment of scars on the eye. Not forgetting that serious traumatising accidents and operations leave not only physical but often mental scars as well.

Therapy with information from the body's natural oscillations or positive external oscillations can have a beneficial effect on the **functioning of organs and tissue**. If we accept the theory that biochemical organ functions are all regulated by a super-ordinate electromagnetic field then it is easy to imagine that appropriate therapeutic effects can be achieved by modulating this oscillating field in a positive manner. Every tissue and every organ has its own specific frequency spectrum. A diseased organ oscillates differently from a healthy one. It also makes a difference, from the point of view of oscillations, whether there is an acute infection, chronic inflammation, auto-immune reaction, poisoning, degenerative process or a malignant degeneration. Viruses, bacteria, fungi and parasites can also alter frequency patterns. Every pathological process on every organ has its inherent oscillation spectrum. Finding these frequency ranges and thereby generating the appropriate counter impulse is a matter of pure empirical research and laborious detailed work.

The Bicom 2000 has about 400 different frequency-based modulation options. The Bicom Optima has an additional 140 in the low frequency range. This gives a large number of treatment options for the most commonly occurring indications. Another option for therapy is to use organ ampoules. These contain positive information from healthy organ functions. They are applied via the Bicom device and can improve the metabolic processes which are still functioning. The improvement in laboratory parameters following Bicom therapy can actually be seen.

We have recorded cases of transaminase (liver enzymes) levels reverting to normal in liver disease and improved creatinine values in patients with kidney failure. An improvement in the parameters of thyroid hormones was also observed.

Meridian therapy is one of the oldest therapy options. As explained earlier, the bioresonance method evolved from electroacupuncture and this in turn developed from

How the bioresonance method functions

traditional Chinese medicine which dates back thousands of years. According to the beliefs of the ancient Chinese, vital energy Chi flows throughout the body in ordered pathways. These 'energy channels' were translated into 'meridians' similar to the orientation lines on the globe. They do not correspond to any clearly defined anatomical structure and cannot be found when the body is dissected. Consequently the existence of these meridians is generally disputed by conventional medicine. Experiments at university hospitals have shown however that a radioactive substance injected into certain acupuncture points spreads along these hypothetical meridians. Electrically charged large molecules in the connective tissue possibly play an important part in relaying information. Some meridian pathways appear to follow the fibres of our autonomic nervous system. The meridians connect a series of acupuncture points.

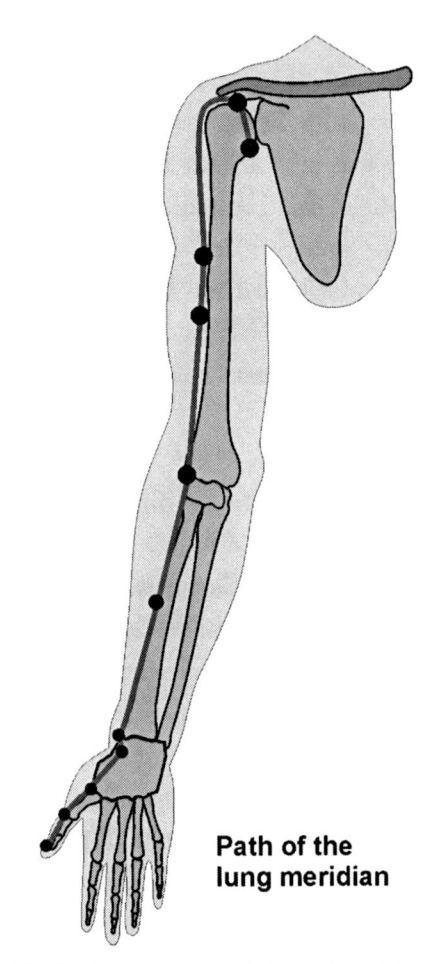

Path of the lung meridian

Fig. 11: Acupuncture points are linked by energy channels known as meridians.

Histological tests were able to show that high concentrations of vegetative nerve fibres can be found at a number of classic acupuncture points. This could also explain the remote action of many acupuncture points through spinal reflexes and feedback from the brain. Stimulating a point (e.g. large intestine 4) on the back of the hand can relieve headache and blocked nose. According to ancient Chinese beliefs the body is healthy if energy flows smoothly and harmoniously through all its organs and tissues. If energy builds up in certain meridians and is deficient in others, symptoms can occur. The disturbed energy path can be diverted and the course of diseases thereby favourably influenced by stimulating certain acupuncture points through needling (acupuncture), massage (acupressure) and, more recently, also by laser or bioresonance treatment.

Measuring the skin's resistance at acupuncture points using electroacupuncture can also be used as a diagnostic tool to indicate the energy in the acupuncture meridians. Classic acupuncture

How the bioresonance method functions

theory describes 14 principal meridians (often named after organs) which can be assigned to five elements or transformation stages (wood, fire, earth, metal and water). Chinese five element theory is very complicated and requires years of experience. But don't worry! It isn't necessary to study Chinese medicine for years in order to work with bioresonance. Through energetic testing and a few ground rules some important therapy principles can be easily yet very effectively implemented with bioresonance.

In practice the start and/or end points of the meridians are usually stimulated for the purposes of **meridian flooding**. Here too each meridian, depending on its current energetic state, has a specific frequency spectrum by which it can be influenced. Another option is to use meridian or element ampoules whose frequency patterns can be applied directly for therapy.

Bioresonance therapy has gained a reputation as a means of effective allergy therapy. Word of the inexplicable yet amazing success has spread rapidly. Many patients sought alternative therapies for their allergic conditions and in the mid 1990s many health insurance funds even bore the cost of this treatment. Of course, that immediately aroused critics and opponents. Some medical and allergy patient groups tried to make this drug-free therapy the object of ridicule for "something which cannot be explained cientifically in the light of current knowledge cannot possibly exist." This hasn't deterred patients however and now hundreds of thousands of people have been relieved of their allergies by bioresonance therapy.

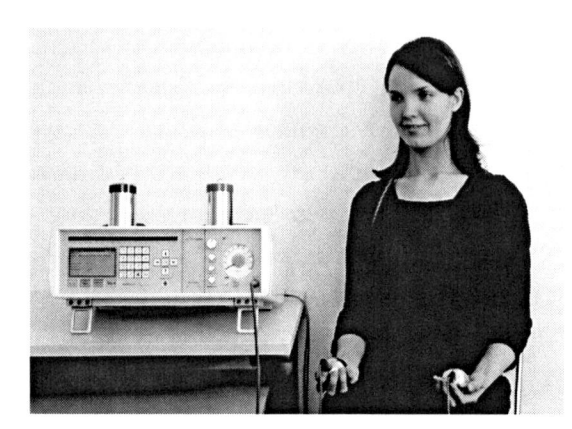

Fig. 12: Allergy therapy with the Bicom bioresonance device.

There are two aspects to bioresonance allergy therapy. The aim is, firstly, to reduce the **allergic diathesis,** i.e. the readiness of the organism to develop allergies and, secondly, to directly eliminate the reaction to the most important allergens. When treating allergy directly, the substance triggering the allergy is usually placed in the input cup. The cup electrode picks up the frequency patterns of the allergen. These are modulated (e.g. inverted) in the Bicom device and applied to the body as a therapeutic impulse using the magnetic field modulation mat and/or spherical metal electrodes. And what happens now? After a few therapy sessions the astonished patient notices that no symptoms occur on contact with the known allergen. It's not difficult to imagine that many individuals first have to absorb this and find it hard to believe or accept.

Biophysical explanatory models obviously now exist for this phenomenon. The theory was initially postulated that the counter oscillation of therapy cancels out the original oscillation of the allergen in the organism due to interference. This deletion of oscillations does actually take place but only while the therapy device is switched on. It cannot explain the prolonged absence of symptoms in allergy patients.

The assumption is now generally held that the allergen information in the organism is stored in the water clusters described earlier. Targeted frequency therapy causes the clusters to be disbanded or modified and the pathogenic information overridden. In 1991 the author introduced into the bioresonance method an additional proven method for treating allergy using acupuncture meridians. It was modelled on a discovery by the kinesiologist J. Scott. He demonstrated that, after flooding certain meridians, tolerance of an allergen concentrated on certain parts of the body increases.

As well as eliminating the main allergens, allergic diathesis should always be treated. The reason for the increasing occurrence of allergies is still disputed in conventional medicine. This is probably a multi-factorial phenomenon. Therapists practising holistically believe that, in addition to genetic factors, diet and increasing environmental contamination play a large part.

Our immune system has adapted over millions of years to the challenges of its environment. The dramatic increase in adverse influences over the past 40 years has led to our immune system becoming overstretched and seemingly reacting in an illogical and uncontrolled fashion. Why do the nasal mucous membranes react to completely harmless birch pollen by sneezing instead of performing their true role of warding off viruses and bacteria? Allergies represent dysregulation of the immune system. Our immune system is a highly complex entity consisting of billions of cells, antibodies and other structures. Holistic therapists believe that chemicals, toxins, some food additives, chronic infections with viruses, bacteria, fungi and parasites, post-vaccinal complications, non-

How the bioresonance method functions

tolerated dental material, radiation exposure and the body's own foci and interference fields, physical and emotional stress overload the immune system and can encourage the occurrence of allergies. Many of these factors can be reduced and neutralised with the bioresonance method, consequently relieving the immune system.

Elimination of toxins and pathogens is also within the domain of bioresonance therapy. In practice the procedure is similar to allergy therapy. Test and therapy ampoules are used which contain the relevant information applied materially or non-materially. This possibly achieves two effects. The body's tolerance threshold to the toxic substance is increased. The organism is better able to compensate for the adverse influence and the (defensive) symptoms decline or disappear. At the same time the organism is stimulated to eliminate these substances more quickly from the body. A marked improvement in patients' symptoms is actually observed. Headaches vanish once amalgam is eliminated, chronic inflammation of the paranasal sinuses improves once wood preservatives are eliminated, neurological symptoms subside once insecticides are eliminated. The list could go on and on.

Due to the latest computer technology it is now also possible to use substances stored digitally instead of test and therapy ampoules. For example **Multisoft** is a computer program which stores over 6000 substances digitally such as allergens, toxins, pathogens as well as homeopathic and allopathic medicines, orthomolecular substances and flower essences. A laptop is placed next to the bioresonance device which copies over the information from these substances to the device input for testing or treating the patient.

Effective **immune modulation** is also possible with the bioresonance method. Firstly the immune system is already relieved as a result of the elimination of chronic adverse influences described above. Secondly, it is possible to increase the immune response by applying appropriate frequency patterns directly. This can reduce susceptibility to infection and diminish the tendency to allergies and auto-immune response. This form of therapy is also very helpful for supporting the immune system during treatments such as chemotherapy and radiotherapy which weaken the immune system. The side-effects of these treatments are noticeably reduced.

The effect of bioresonance therapy on the **hormone system** is also impressive. Patients (both male and female) who suffer menopausal symptoms such as hot flushes, outbreaks

How the bioresonance method functions

of sweating and depression experience noticeable relief after just a few therapy sessions. Hormone preparations are often no longer necessary. Hormonally induced migraine, menstrual disorders, problems following pregnancy and in puberty can be treated. A number of 'Bicom babies' have been born following successful treatment of fertility problems.

The **treatment of wounds and injuries** is also a field covered by the bioresonance method. Some dentists and surgeons have bought a Bicom device mainly to treat patients before and after surgery. Reports agree that wounds heal more quickly and healing is hardly ever impaired. Consumption of antibiotics and painkillers has fallen rapidly and haematoma and swellings subside faster. Secondary healing or scar interference fields very rarely occur. Bioresonance is also used in **sports medicine**. Injuries heal more quickly and, in competitive sport, a number of Olympic teams are now looked after by bioresonance therapists.

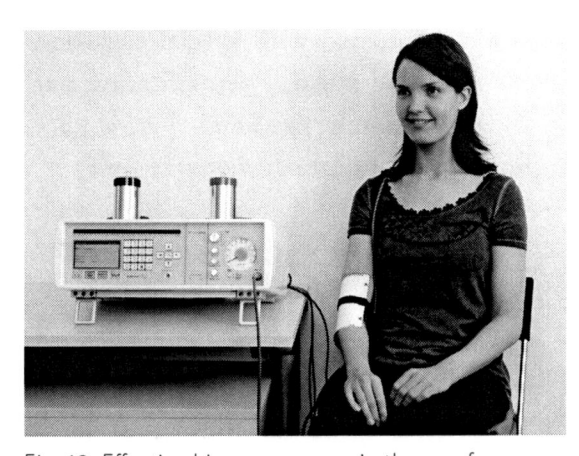

Fig. 13: Effective bioresonance pain therapy for epicondylitis (tennis elbow).

Pain therapy with the bioresonance method is gaining in importance. Acute pain can often be rapidly reduced. Improvements have been achieved with chronic pain where other methods have been exhausted. Bioresonance has also proved effective in combination with other methods of pain therapy. Indications are migraine, headaches, blocks in the temporomandibular joint, back pain, osteoarthritis and arthritis in the large and small joints, tennis elbow and carpal tunnel syndrome. A Turkish neurosurgeon was able to save patients from surgery on the intervertebral disks by using bioresonance.[11]

There are also examples of supportive treatment with bioresonance in **cancer treatment**. It can be used to accompany other treatment such as chemotherapy and radiotherapy. Here programs are used for pre- and post-operative treatment, elimination of scar interference, removal of radiation contamination and to detoxify and stabilise the

---

[11] Dr. Kiran, Kongress des Internationalen Medizinischen Arbeitskreises BRT [International Congress of the Medical Research Group BRT], April 2007 Fulda.

immune system. Test and therapy ampoules are also used which, amongst other things, contain the information from tumour tissue as well as that from the surrounding healthy tissue. The aim is to encourage 'apoptosis', the controlled death of the tumour cells and to improve the functioning of healthy tissue. Through this treatment the side-effects of aggressive therapies can be reduced and the patient's quality of life improved. No studies are available yet on the effect of bioresonance over the course of cancer however countless observations made of individual cases give reason to hope.

Anti-smoking therapy is a combination of programs for organ regeneration, detoxification and to support the autonomic nervous system. It is probably the only smoking cessation treatment which also detoxifies the body at the same time. The craving for cigarettes subsides and withdrawal symptoms are largely reduced. Grateful patients often pass on the recommendation to relatives and work colleagues. For some practices this indication was a simple and lucrative way into the bioresonance method.

In **weight loss therapy** ear acupuncture points are stimulated with special electrodes through bioresonance programs for metabolism, hormone system, detoxification and autonomic nervous system. Combined with an appropriately modified diet, a good sustained weight loss can be achieved while improving metabolism at the same time.

> The bioresonance method can have a beneficial effect on a number of acute and chronic diseases. Considerable positive experience of treatment for radiation exposure, scar interference fields and supporting organ and meridian disturbance is available. Allergies and also the chronic adverse effects of toxins and pathogens can be treated using the bioresonance method. The immune system and hormone system are stabilised. The bioresonance method is also used in sports medicine, pain therapy, cancer therapy and treatment of addiction.

On the trail of hidden causes of disease

Biophysical test methods

Thorough diagnosis by conventional medical techniques is an important and essential requirement before using an alternative method of treatment. In most cases this diagnosis describes the clinical picture but does not reveal the actual causes of the condition. Chronic enteritis, for example, can be diagnosed by laboratory tests, X-ray, endoscopy with histology and treatment generally tends to be symptomatic.

Biophysical test methods, as they are known, enable us to discover valuable information about causes or factors affecting the deterioration of a patient's condition beyond the boundaries of conventional medical diagnosis. Perhaps food intolerance, infection with fungi, bacteria, viruses or parasites, toxin contamination with heavy metals or chemicals, radiation exposure or the body's natural interference fields play a part in this enteritis?

Biophysical treatment of these harmful factors often produces a dramatic improvement in the course of the affected patient's condition. As with diagnosis by conventional medical methods, the quality of biophysical test results depends to a large extent upon the training, competence and experience of the therapist. It is not (yet) possible to examine and assess these methods according to currently valid scientific standards since therapy always consists of the therapist's individual measures. What ultimately counts is that treatment is successful. This proves that the test conducted earlier was correct. The most common biophysical test methods are Dr Voll's electroacupuncture, the kinesiological muscle test, pulse diagnosis and the resonance test with the tensor.

As described earlier, the bioresonance method was developed from **Voll's electroacupuncture (EAV)**. In classic EAV skin resistance is measured at over 300 acupuncture points with a test stylus. These include almost all the points of the classic acupuncture meridians from Traditional Chinese Medicine. Dr Voll also discovered a whole series of similar points on the body and assigned them to new Voll's acupuncture meridians according to their function. So, in this system, there is an allergy, nervous system and organ degeneration meridian, amongst others. The start and end points of

On the trail of hidden causes of diseases

all traditional and Voll's meridians are located on the corner of the nailbeds of the fingers and toes.

Measuring these hand and foot points is generally sufficient to enable bioresonance therapists to diagnose factors affecting the patient's energy and to determine appropriate therapy. The energetic connections discovered by Dr Voll between meridians and teeth are also interesting. As a result, Chinese five element theory has been extended by the addition of important diagnostic criteria. Reproducible test results are obtained if the skin's moisture levels and the pressure of the measuring stylus are accurate. Test readings are indicated by the needle's deflection on the scale of the measuring device. A scale reading of 50 indicates a normal energy level at the acupuncture point. Scale readings above 60 and below 40 point to disturbed energy levels

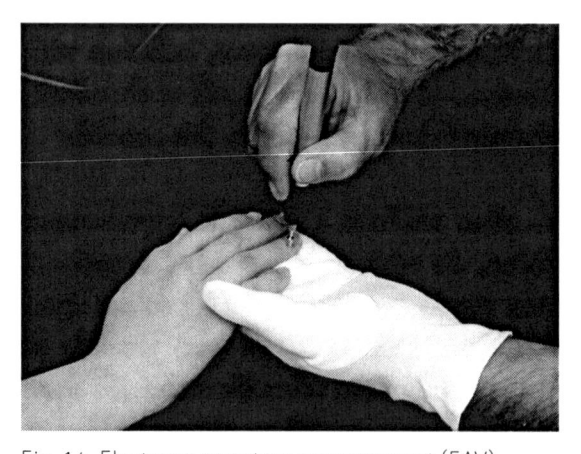

Fig. 14: Electroacupuncture measurement (EAV).

Substances introduced into the measuring circuit which shift the scale reading towards 50 can be considered as medication for this patient. Toxic substances, pathogens and allergens are only imported into the measuring circuit after being physically inverted by the Bicom device (see above). If the needle is deflected towards 50, these substances are regarded as having an adverse effect on energy and generally need to be treated.

Kinesiology comes from the Greek 'study of movement'. It deals with testing and correcting impaired muscle function. It is fascinating for patients to experience how muscle strength and tone alter under certain conditions. Therapists usually work with the upper arm muscle (deltoid) in practice. The patient holds the arm outstretched forwards or to the side. The therapist now attempts to push the arm downwards by applying gentle pressure while the patient is told to resist. If the patient also comes into contact with information which adversely affects energy levels (allergen, toxin, germ), then muscle tone is reduced and the arm becomes weaker under the same pressure.

On the trail of hidden causes of diseases

Many patients (and therapists) only believe this when they have experienced it on their own bodies. If, for example, the arm becomes much weaker than before on contact with a milk ampoule, this can be regarded as allergy or intolerance of dairy products. If the previously existing symptoms are reduced or disappear after introducing a milk-free diet, this confirms the energetic diagnosis was correct.

Energetic diagnosis is only a small part of kinesiology however. The energy flow in the body can be balanced and the body's powers of self-healing stimulated by appropriate kinesiological exercises. There are reports that the ancient Greeks and the Incas evidently used muscle tests for medical purposes.

Kinesiology was rediscovered and systematically investigated in the 1960s by the chiropractor George Goodheart. Since then kinesiology has enjoyed success throughout the world. There are institutes and training establishments in a number of countries which disseminate this method for therapists and also a lay audience. In the context of bioresonance, kinesiological testing is used in particular to test adverse influences and determine appropriate therapy programs.

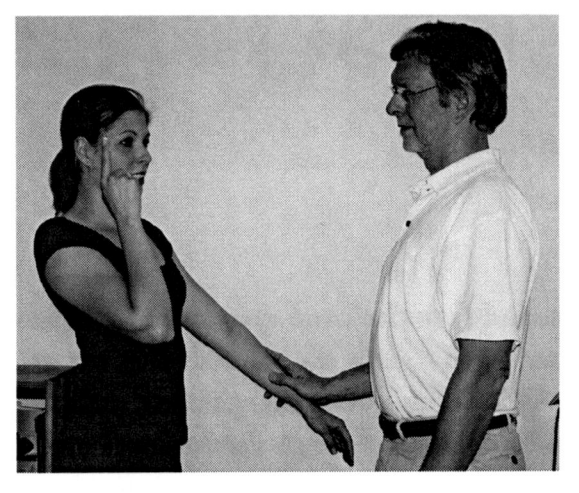

Fig. 15: Kinesiological muscle test.

Pulse testing was already used as a diagnostic method in Traditional Chinese Medicine. It is used in a modified form in ear acupuncture in the reticulo auricular reflex (RAC) discovered by Nogier. We are not talking here of pulse rate or heart rate but about pulse quality, such as pressure and rhythmic inflow and outflow. Changes in pulse quality following the influence of detrimental factors or medication give the experienced therapist important diagnostic information on how to proceed with treatment.

The **tensor** is a physical instrument for detecting resonance phenomena. It consists of a handle, a wire and a sensor element. This can take the shape of a ring, a ball, a spiral or a small satellite dish (as with the BiRek tensor electrode). Using the tensor the experienced therapist can decide whether resonance or dissonance exists between two information fields (e.g. patient and substance or patient and output of the Bicom device). If the tensor moves from side to side this indicates a positive resonance phenomenon, while if it moves up and down there is no resonance. The patient can be tested thoroughly and directly with this method but even testing a drop of the patient's blood provides results which are useful for therapy.

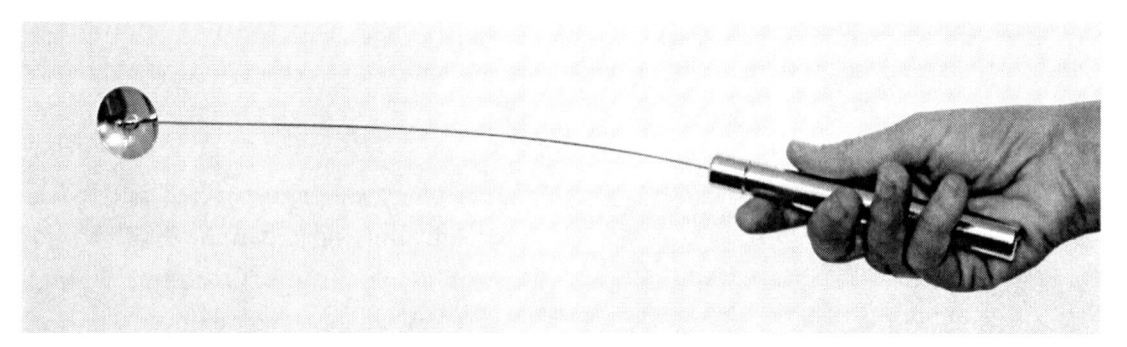

Fig. 16: The resonance test can be performed with the tensor.

Energy-based diagnostic methods are continuously criticised and questioned by representatives of conventional medicine. The situation as regards clinical trials does not yet permit scientific validity. What are we actually measuring with energetic test methods and why do they sometimes agree with results obtained through conventional medicine and sometimes not? We are determining whether the electromagnetic (or other?) oscillatory field resonates with the oscillatory field of a substance (allergen, toxin, test ampoule, nosode, medicine) or of therapeutic information (Bicom device). This is the case if the same or similar information is present in the body or oscillatory field of the patient. A conventional medical diagnosis cannot always be derived from this.

If the liver tests as weak, for example, it is not clear whether there is actually a clinical disorder. Is it fatty degeneration of the liver, cirrhosis, hepatitis or perhaps just inadequate capacity to eliminate or a functional disorder resulting from misguided emotions? The results of energetic testing must always be interpreted while taking into account the patient's medical history, a physical examination, lab readings and other results. In no way does it replace the need for conventional medical diagnosis. The test result is particularly important for the resulting energetic therapy with bioresonance, homeopathy or other holistic method.

On the trail of hidden causes of diseases

Another example: the energetic test result reveals infestation with parasites. Here too there are different possible interpretations: 1. The parasite is actually physically present; 2. The parasite itself is no longer in the body but has left behind traces in the form of toxins, metabolites or just purely non-material electromagnetic information; 3. This parasite is not and never was in the body but, owing to other adverse influences, the patient has an oscillation pattern which closely resembles that of this parasite. In the first case a conventional blood test or stool examination can often confirm this result unless the parasite has hidden away in the tissue and cannot be tracked down.

If the parasitic infestation is severe, allopathic medication may be necessary but, if it is a mild attack, bioresonance therapy is often sufficient. This probably reduces the parasite's vitality and strengthens the body's natural defence system so that it can easily be eliminated. In the second and third case there will be a marked discrepancy between energetic testing and conventional medical diagnosis.

If material or non-material traces of the parasite still exist, elimination follows the principle of **isopathy** – treating a condition with the exact same substance that causes it. For bioresonance therapy a test ampoule of the same parasite is applied or a nosode is administered. Nosodes are dilutions of pathogens potentiated according to homeopathic or isopathic guidelines. In the third case a resonance pattern of unclear origin exists in the patient without parasites or their traces being present. Here treatment follows the **homeopathic** principle – like is treated with like [the substance producing the most similar symptoms in healthy individuals to those experienced by the patient is used for treatment.] Treatment with the counter oscillation or nosode remains the same. The patient will benefit from treatment with bioresonance and/or nosodes in all three cases. The symptoms generally improve noticeably.

When testing toxins and heavy metals, interpretation is subject to the same criteria. For example, mercurious solubilis (mercury) is used both isopathically to help eliminate mercury poisoning and homeopathically to treat symptoms which resemble those of mercury poisoning. Classic homeopathy recognises many substances whose oscillation potential is used to treat a wide variety of diseases without the symptoms being directly connected with the substance. Potentiated arnica is a good homeopathic remedy for injuries which definitely have nothing to do with arnica poisoning.

On the trail of hidden causes of diseases

When testing allergens and (food) intolerance the energetic test indicates whether the body's oscillatory system is burdened by these substances or reacts to them with (visible or hidden) symptoms. It is of no significance whether this is a genuine allergy, a pseudo-allergy or an intolerance. The patient benefits, in any event, from the abstention from the substance and from having these thoroughly tested allergens treated. This situation explains, however, the problems encountered with comparing conventional medical tests and energetic testing. This issue will be examined in more detail in the chapter 'Effectiveness and evidence'.

An experienced holistic therapist will take note of the findings obtained through conventional medicine and incorporate them into his therapeutic deliberations. As a rule, bioresonance therapy is mainly based on the results of the therapist's own energetic testing however.

There is another problem: energetic testing is susceptible to disruption. But we are familiar with this from conventional medicine. Listening to the heart sounds, measuring blood pressure and other physical examinations as well as ultrasound and interpreting X-rays does not always produce exactly the same findings with different doctors. Medicine is not an exact science like physics and chemistry. We have learnt to live with this uncertainty and range of variation and it only plays a relatively minor role in a doctor's daily routine.

This applies perhaps to an even greater degree to energetic test methods. Energy fields beyond the patient, as well as the therapist's energy field, may influence the result of the test. Experienced therapists will remove any possible sources of energetic interference, such as large pieces of jewellery, quartz watches, mobile phones, magnetic or electrical equipment, etc., from the patient and the test area. The therapist's thoughts which alter his own energy field can also affect the test result.

Fatigue, difficulty in concentration and one's own physical and emotional blocks may have just as negative an effect as unclear intentions, partiality, doubt, prejudice or stress of the test. The stress of a test situation may influence the test result which is why double blind trials often do not work and are not advised.

Curiosity about the diagnosis, openness, the wish to help the patient, concentration and a clear intention without expecting a particular result are the best prerequisites for good

On the trail of hidden causes of diseases

and usable results. No particular mental abilities are necessary. Virtually anyone can learn the methods of energetic testing; prior medical knowledge is not even required. It is important however to have good sound training and to keep practising. Experienced therapists definitely score over 90% when it comes to testing correctly. A little self-criticism does no harm however: a result of one hundred percent is impossible in conventional or alternative medicine.

> Energetic test methods such as Voll's electroacupuncture, the kinesiological muscle test, pulse testing and the resonance test with the tensor give the holistic therapist important diagnostic information about the existence of energetic problems in the patient and help him decide the next step for therapy.

Swift help

Acute disorders

What can be treated with the bioresonance method? It can be inferred from the mode of action that basically all clinical pictures where fully functioning (residual) tissue still exists can be treated. Bioresonance is a regulatory therapy which means that tissue and organs must be capable of regulation or at least of being activated to regulate themselves once more. This shows the limits of the bioresonance method and of all other alternative methods. An organ which is totally destroyed cannot therefore be treated and a missing leg will not grow again. Over the course of the years widely differing experience has been gained with a broad range of clinical pictures. A selection of the most important treatable health disorders is presented in the following chapters using case studies from daily practice.

According to the principles described in the previous chapters, bioresonance obviously has an anti-allergic effect inhibiting inflammation, modulating the immune system and relieving pain. It has a positive effect on both acute clinical pictures and chronic disorders. In acute health disorders the effect is usually felt immediately by the patient and observed directly by the therapist. This includes acute infections of the respiratory tract such as colds, flu, bronchitis and inflammation of the middle ear as well as acute gastrointestinal infection and urinary infection.

The symptoms and patient's general state of health are observed to improve rapidly and the illness is less prolonged. Programs with the body's natural information (electrodes on diseased organ) and pathological bodily secretions (sputum, stool, urine) are used. If the germ which is responsible is known or has been thoroughly tested, the appropriate test ampoule for bacteria or viruses can be used in therapy.

Here is a case study by Dr. med. W.-D. K.: an 18-year-old man presented with **acute bronchitis**: cough, temperature of 39.5° and, on examination, rhonchal noises on the lungs. After one session of bioresonance therapy the patient's temperature rose to 40.5° and he just wanted to sleep. The next morning his temperature had dropped to 37.5°, he had slept right though the night and felt as fit as a fiddle. There was no need for

Swift help

conventional medicines such as antibiotics.

Inflammation which is not caused by germs generally also responds well to the bioresonance method. Here is an example from my own personal experience: after a strenuous game of badminton I suddenly experienced violent pain in my right elbow. I could scarcely bend my arm, typical for **acute tennis elbow** (epicondylitis). I knew from past practice that treatment often lasted many weeks and months. My wife treated me with the bioresonance device straight away. At first the symptoms worsened for a few hours. The next morning all the pain had disappeared and I was able to play badminton again.

There are also a large number of positive reports of the treatment of wounds and injuries. A 34-year-old patient consulted non-medical practitioner I. Ph with **acute torn calf muscle fibre**. An orthopaedic specialist had diagnosed the condition and prescribed six weeks' rest. The rather impatient patient decided to try bioresonance therapy. The pain had disappeared after just one treatment session and the patient felt so good that she went to a dance the next day.

It's no surprise that sports physicians are looking into this means of treatment. The bioresonance device has already accompanied a number of professional teams to the Olympic Games.

Surgeons and dentists are also exploiting the ability of bioresonance to relieve pain, reduce swelling and promote regeneration to prepare patients for surgery or in post-operative treatment. They are in agreement that, as a result, infected wounds or secondary healing rarely occur. Haematoma and oedema are broken down more quickly and consumption of analgesics or antibiotics is significantly reduced.

Dr. med. P.-G. V. reports of a 56-year-old patient with **acute lumbago** with loss of neurological function. In addition to considerable pain the patient experienced loss of sensory and motor function and was no longer able to walk. A CT scan confirmed a **slipped disk** and the orthopaedic surgeon wanted to operate immediately. The patient refused surgery and tried conservative therapy with physiotherapy, chiropractic medicine and stimulation current but to no avail. Bioresonance therapy altered the situation. After a series of treatment sessions over seven days, the patient's condition initially deteriorated briefly before improving dramatically. Feeling suddenly returned in the little toe and then, after a short time, the other neurological symptoms regressed. After five days the patient was symptom-free and able to walk and work again. Surgery was no longer necessary.

> Bioresonance therapy is effective for all acute and chronic disorders provided that existing tissue is still capable of regulation. Rapid success with acute bronchitis, tennis elbow, wounds, injuries and slipped disk is reported.

The new widespread disease

Allergic disorders group

The bioresonance method has become well-known for its ability to treat allergies swiftly and effectively. Word of its obvious success has spread rapidly amongst patients and consequently many allergy sufferers are seeking out the practices of bioresonance therapists. This is certainly attributable to the fact that the number of people suffering from allergies has been steadily increasing for years and many patients are disappointed in the options available in conventional medicine.

Billions are being invested in allergy research and knowledge about our immune system and the mechanisms which trigger allergic reactions is increasing continually. Yet so far this has had little practical impact on patients. In most cases allergies are treated in the same way today as they were 30 years ago. Either the patient is recommended to avoid the allergen (something which is often easier said than done) or the symptoms are suppressed by means of drugs. But antihistamines and cortisone preparations only help the patient while they are taken. They have no effect on the cause of the symptoms. Specific immune therapy (hyposensitisation) is only possible with a small number of allergens. It generally involves considerable outlay of time and money, does not always help and the risk of side-effects cannot be ignored.

So it is no surprise that an increasing number of patients are seeking alternatives. It is astonishing that, despite the large number of reports of success and a series of positive scientific studies, 'official' conventional medicine ignores this means of treatment. It is precisely the allergic disorders group and the medical and economic challenges they bring where one would think that science and politics would be eager for effective new methods. But other interests obviously play a part here. It is left up to the patients themselves to search for a glimmer of hope.

The bioresonance method has demonstrated considerable success with well-known allergic disorders such as skin rashes (eczema, skin eruptions), allergic rhinitis and sinusitis, hay fever, allergy to animal hair, bronchial asthma, allergic gastro-intestinal disorders and food allergies. Experience has shown that allergic reactions play a part in

The new widespread disease

a range of other clinical pictures which are not categorised as classic allergic disorders. Here too there is evidence of successful treatment following appropriate testing and therapy. This includes neurodermatitis, colitis, cystitis, cardiac irregularity, headaches, fibromyalgia, poor concentration and chronic fatigue syndrome. Viewed in the widest sense, the allergic disorders group also includes autoimmune disorders (thyroiditis, colitis, multiple sclerosis) and these can also often be treated with positive results.

Symptoms of allergic disorders

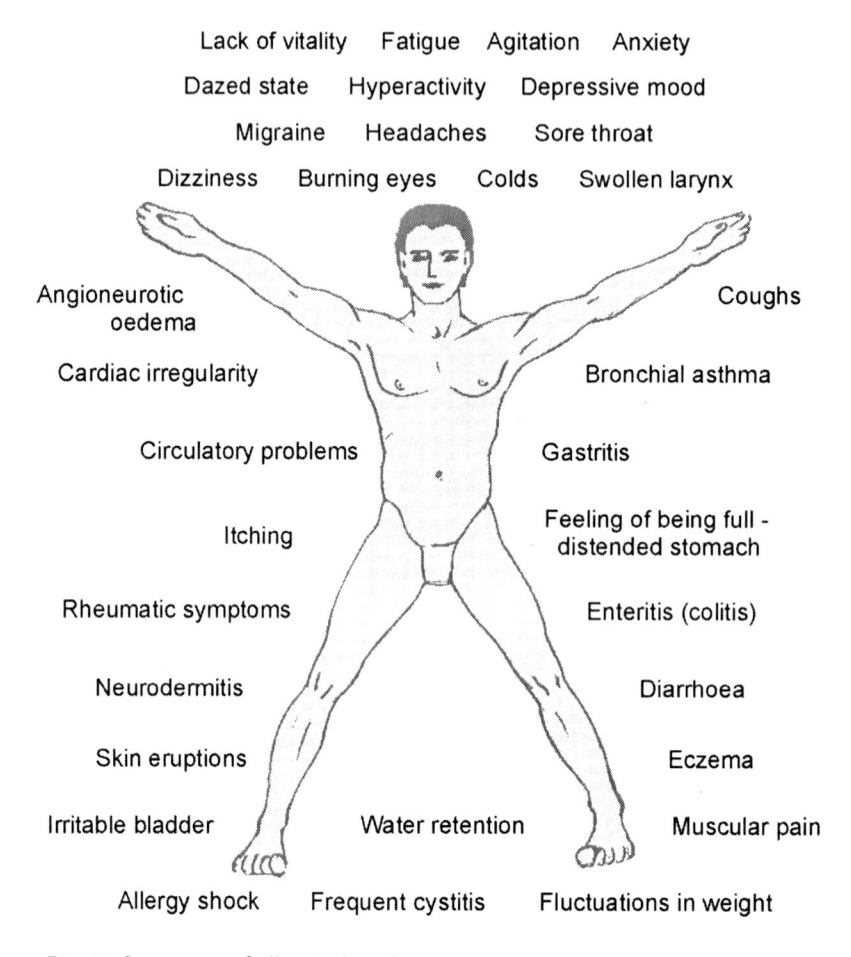

Lack of vitality Fatigue Agitation Anxiety
Dazed state Hyperactivity Depressive mood
Migraine Headaches Sore throat
Dizziness Burning eyes Colds Swollen larynx

Angioneurotic oedema
Cardiac irregularity
Circulatory problems
Itching
Rheumatic symptoms
Neurodermitis
Skin eruptions
Irritable bladder
Allergy shock

Water retention
Frequent cystitis

Coughs
Bronchial asthma
Gastritis
Feeling of being full - distended stomach
Enteritis (colitis)
Diarrhoea
Eczema
Muscular pain
Fluctuations in weight

Fig. 17: Symptoms of allergic disorders

Different approaches to treating allergy have developed in bioresonance therapy. This often consists of a combination of treating the individual allergens and treating the overall disposition for allergy (allergic diathesis). Once a troublesome allergen (e.g. pollen, mould, house dust, animal hair) has been treated, the patient very quickly notices their symptoms improve. Therapy blocks, disease foci, radiation exposure, toxic contamination from heavy metals or chemicals and chronic infections from fungi, viruses, bacteria or parasites often play a part in the treatment of allergic diathesis. Chronic food allergies which often go unnoticed by the patient are particularly important.

Cows' milk and wheat intolerance are a common feature. The body's disposition for allergy can often be improved to such an extent simply by treating these two principal allergens that 'lesser' allergies no longer need treating at all.

> Allergic disorders are assuming ever greater significance in today's world. The bioresonance method is very successful with all the conditions in the allergic disorders group.

From hay fever to asthma

Respiratory tract diseases

When the subject of allergy is raised, many people immediately think of patients with a runny nose, sneezing, itchy eyes and shortness of breath. The respiratory tract is indeed the most common target organ of acute and chronic allergic reactions. Symptoms range in intensity from slight itchiness in the nose through hay fever and chronic sinusitis to life-threatening bronchial asthma.

Classic allergy testing predominantly seeks out the inhalational allergens such as house dust mites, moulds, animal hair, pollen and fragrances. The bioresonance therapist will not only search for the allergens triggering these symptoms but will also seek out and treat fundamental energetic disorders such as chronic food allergies, chronic toxic contamination and therapy blocks. Children and those who have only been suffering for a short period can often be completely cleared of their symptoms with bioresonance therapy. A complete recovery is not always possible in older asthmatics who have had the condition for some time. However even these patients often experience some relief from their symptoms and an improvement in their quality of life. As a result long-term medication can usually be reduced.

A further advantage of the bioresonance method is that there is no need to avoid the allergens responsible during and after therapy. It is not necessary to convert the bedroom into a dust-free operating room or to give away the much-loved family pet.

When he was seven months old, little Hannes first contracted **spastic bronchitis**, mostly combined with infections. His asthma attacks became increasingly frequent. At this time he also began suffering from a chronic blocked nose and itching eczema on his hand. He was receiving conventional medical treatment and each day had to inhale medicines containing disodium chromoglycate (DSCG) which only brought a slight improvement however.

At the age of four Hannes came to our practice with his mother. Kinesiological testing revealed allergy to cows' milk, white flour, house dust mites and severe infestation with mould.

From hay fever to asthma

First the cows' milk allergy was treated twice with the bioresonance device, then the wheat allergy once. In addition programs for eliminating toxins and activating metabolism were used.

A perceptible improvement could already be seen after these first three therapy sessions alone. Hannes was able to breathe deeply and freely once more and the eczema on his hand had disappeared. The daily inhalations were no longer necessary. Four bioresonance therapy sessions followed at weekly intervals at which the house dust allergy and mould infestation were treated. A total of seven therapy sessions were needed over the course of two months. After this Hannes was completely free of symptoms, as he was six years later.

For many patients it is initially disconcerting to be asked to bring 'original material' with them to their next therapy session. For until then they have only known tests with prefabricated allergen extracts and treatment with corresponding medication. Experience has shown that reactions to different types of dust, moulds of differing origin or the hairs of different breeds of animal actually vary widely. There are patients who react allergically to poodles and dachshunds but not to boxers or sheepdogs.

Bioresonance is an information-based therapy. The more closely the therapy information matches the information triggering the allergy, the better the results of therapy. So the patient brings some dust from the vacuum cleaner bag, mould from the bathroom or hair from their own moggy as well as from their grandma's, neighbours' and classmates' cats.

Daniel came to us for treatment at the age of thirteen. He had been suffering from bronchial asthma since he was seven and was continuously reliant on medication. Three years' hyposensitisation to house dust brought little relief. When a small young cat joined the family, his respiratory problems got even worse. The paediatrician commented that the cat would probably have to go to an animal shelter. To which his little brother retorted: "I'd rather Daniel went to a children's home than the cat to an animal shelter." Both were able to stay at home. Daniel was treated with the bioresonance method for wheat, Candida albicans, house dust, mould, mercury and cat hair.

Fifteen years later his mother came back to the practice on another matter. She reported that her son was now grown up and working in Munich and had not experienced any

From hay fever to asthma

further allergic symptoms since that treatment.

Successful treatment of **allergy to animal hairs** is one of the most gratifying jobs of a therapist. (Virtually) all doctors tell their patients that their four-legged friends have to go. Dramatic family scenes have apparently already been played out. In most cases patients were able to keep their pets; the symptoms no longer appeared on contact with animals. A miracle for many patients and a scientific puzzle for many medical colleagues.

Allergies to dogs, cats, rabbits, hamsters, guineapigs, horses, rats and mice, budgerigars and parrots have been successfully treated in our practice. We treated a woman for camel hair allergy so that she could join a camel riding holiday in India and an animal keeper at the zoo for monkey hair allergy. We desensitised a number of employees of a pharmaceutical company who worked in the animal laboratory to overcome their allergy to the hairs of rats and mice from the lab.

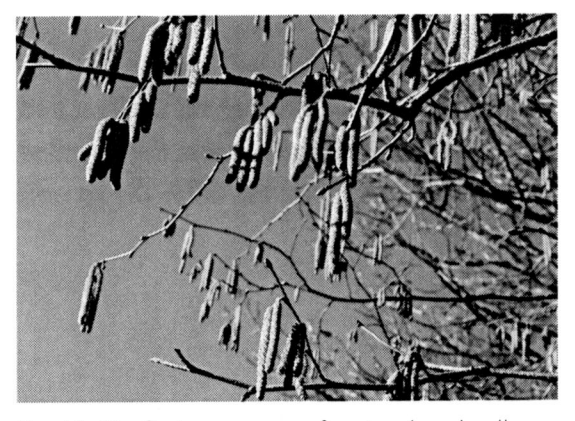

Fig. 18: The first annoyance of spring: hazel pollen.

Pollen allergy is a growing problem each year. More and more people are affected and the symptoms are becoming increasingly more violent. Over 20% of all Germans now suffer from hay fever. The 'change in level' is a particular worry. What starts with itching eyes and the impulse to sneeze can end in violent bronchial asthma after a few years. It is precisely this which conventional medicine's hyposensitisation attempts to prevent, although not always successfully. Some allergy specialists do not even bother with it if a large number of different allergens are tested. And having a cortisone injection (or several) every year is not the ideal solution either.

It is not always easy treating hay fever, even for experienced bioresonance therapists. One problem is that most patients don't just react to the 'clean' pollen allergens, the pollen is contaminated with environmental factors such as exhaust gases, airborne particles and pesticides. This explains why the allergen structure of pollen may vary not only from place to place but also from year to year.

We know patients who following a series of bioresonance treatment sessions have been symptom-free for many years. Yet there are others who need booster treatment year after year in spring or summer.

Ideally bioresonance is used as a preventive measure in the winter months, yet it also helps in 'season' with highly acute symptoms. And not just with young people, but also with elderly patients, as the following case shows.

The non-medical practitioner A.K. reports of an 80-year-old patient who came to the practice in spring with an acute pollen allergy. Despite her age the patient was still very active and did not want to take any more medication. She explained that she'd suffered badly from hay fever for 30 years and already tried various therapies. The allergy medication she took affected her general state of health; she felt very tired, weary and weak. Testing revealed severe allergy to early flowering plants, especially hazel.

Following basic therapy, scar interference was removed, toxins eliminated via the liver and the lymph system activated. The actual allergy therapy for hazel pollen was then carried out. The patient already felt much better after the first therapy session. After the second session the following week her symptoms disappeared.[12]

> Respiratory disorders such as chronic sinusitis, pollinosis and bronchial asthma can usually be treated successfully with the bioresonance method. People allergic to animal hair can generally keep their pets.

---

[12] Regumed: Number one p. 4, 1, 2006.

Our largest organ – the skin

Dermatological diseases

Skin disease, especially if it affects the face or other visible parts of the body, is an allergic symptom which is often regarded subjectively as particularly unpleasant. The disorder is impossible to hide from other people and fear of possible contagion may lead some sufferers to withdraw from social contact.

Allergically induced rashes may affect only small areas of the body or extend throughout the whole body. Symptoms range in intensity from slight reddening of the skin through scaly or oozing eczema to ulceration. The symptoms are almost always linked with itching of varying severity. Scratching provides short-term relief but usually aggravates the rash and can lead to additional infections. In conventional medicine a distinction is made between acute or chronic skin eruptions and eczema, neurodermatitis and some other clinical pictures.

Treatment is usually topical; the cause is generally unknown. Cortisone ointment certainly helps but only while it is applied. More long-term success is rare. In our experience rashes may possibly be caused both by external noxious substances and internal factors.

Diagnosis of **contact allergies** is generally less difficult. Following a varying period of exposure to the allergen the typical rash appears on the skin. Examples of this are metal allergies, most frequently nickel and cobalt, allergies to plasters, to natural or synthetic clothing and to fragrances in soaps and detergents. In conventional medicine a patch test is carried out to diagnose the condition. The allergen being tested is applied to the skin for at least 24 hours and a reading then taken of the skin's reaction. This method is simple and reliable yet can set therapists off on the wrong track.

In most cases of neurodermatitis and chronic eczema the cause tends to be internal. The traditional test methods used in conventional medicine are often unable to detect the cause of the symptoms. Consequently it is often disputed whether these are allergic conditions. Genetic disposition cannot be dismissed and a psychological component

Our largest organ - the skin

definitely plays an important part.

Many years of experience by numerous alternative therapists has shown that a chronic (often masked) food allergy to cows' milk or wheat, usually coupled with intestinal mycosis, plays a crucial role in neurodermatitis and chronic eczema.

Diagnosis is often only possible by means of an energetic test method. Neither prick tests (allergen is injected under the skin) nor antibody determination in the blood are reliable here. It is crucial for the therapist and naturally also for the patient that, following abstention and treatment of these allergens, the skin's symptoms improve or even disappear completely. Successful therapy confirms the diagnosis was correct.

Experienced therapists often find other factors such as other foods or food additives, heavy metals and environmental toxins, inoculations and medication, chronic fungal, viral, bacterial or parasitic infections, etc. are also responsible for causing the condition.

The non-medical practitioner M.S. reported on a four-year-old boy with severe neurodermatitis. He fought tooth and nail and vociferously when brought to the practice by his parents. His face, arms and legs were chafed and covered with scabs. The rash was less marked on his trunk yet the boy complained of pain throughout his body. His parents were desperate. They no longer knew what to feed the boy. "For a year he has eaten only sweet dry rice", explained his mother with tears in her eyes.

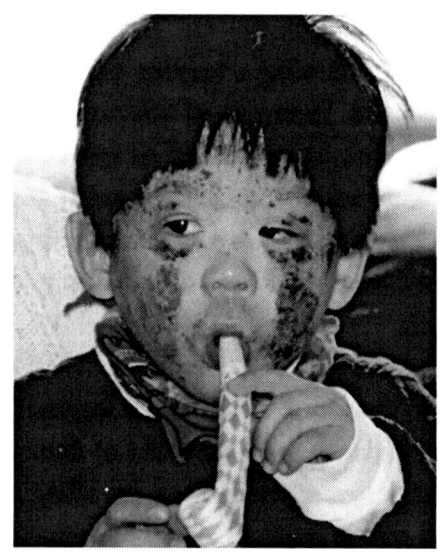

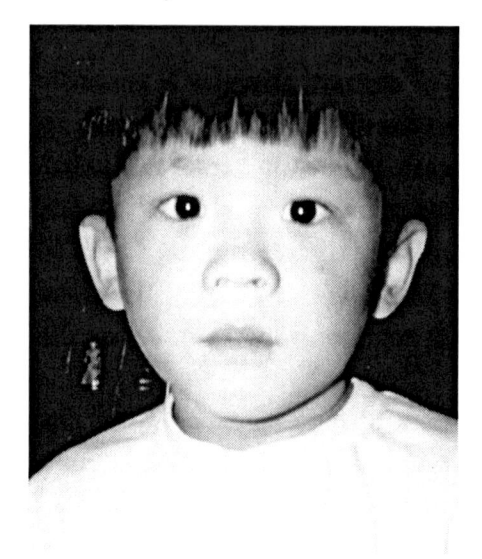

Fig. 19 and 20: Boy with neurodermatitis before and after bioresonance therapy.

Our largest organ - the skin

Electroacupuncture testing revealed several food allergies, mineral deficiencies and contamination with inherited toxins. After just three weeks' allergy therapy with the Bicom device, together with appropriate modifications to the diet and administration of orthomolecular substances, his condition was visibly improved. The little boy now came into the practice laughing. After three further treatment sessions the little boy was absolutely symptom-free. His wounds and scabs had healed completely. The little boy was alert and happy and able to eat everything once more. Three years later no further symptoms had appeared either.[13]

Children generally respond quickly to bioresonance therapy. Treatment is often more difficult and laborious in adults with a long history of the condition. Yet success is possible here too as the following case shows. A 33-year-old woman came to our practice and reported that she had suffered from neurodermatitis since birth. She had already tried several alternative methods of treatment. Her non-medical practitioner treated her with acupuncture, homeopathic remedies and conducted colon cleansing. She had to relieve episodes of neurodermatitis with cortisone ointment.

Her skin had deteriorated markedly following the birth of her son four months earlier. Dry eczema appeared on her face, neck and cleavage as well as on her arms and legs. In spring and summer she also suffered from allergic rhinoconjunctivitis.

Kinesiological testing revealed allergies to cows' milk, wheat, various fruits, coffee, chlorinated water as well as early flowering plants and grass pollen.

Candida mycosis in the intestine and scar interference in the lower abdominal region was also detected. Colon cleansing was performed and the food allergies were treated in eight weekly sessions. Since the patient still evidently reacted to chlorinated water, this was treated again intensively. Over this period the skin had improved considerably. Only a slight rash on the neck and wrists was still visible.

> Numerous cases of neurodermatitis and chronic eczema were successfully treated with the bioresonance method.

---

[13] Regumed: Number one p. 2, 2, 2002.

Problems in the digestive tract

Gastro-intestinal disorders

As we have already repeatedly seen, intestinal function plays a large part in the allergic process. First of all digestive function: from the oral cavity via the stomach to the small intestine the breaking up, selection and absorption of foodstuffs represents the most important task.

The large intestine tends to be responsible for excreting unwanted substances and waste products. In addition it is involved in regulating the vitamin, mineral and water balance in the body. Beneath the intestinal mucous membranes lie large collections of lymph nodes which make up around 70% of our entire immune system. The intestines harbour 10 to 100 billion micro-organisms (that is more cells than all the body's cells put together), which are essential not only for digestive function but also for the immune system to function properly.

Allergy sufferers often display reduced activity of the digestive enzymes, coupled with impaired intestinal mucosal barrier function as well as malfunction of the gut-associated immune system. Large molecules are often not broken down completely and penetrate through the porous intestinal mucous membrane to the lymphatic tissue where an intensified immune response may occur. According to an established theory this is the main cause for the development of food allergies and intolerance. This dysfunction is accompanied by disturbed intestinal flora, i.e. imperfect mix of micro-organisms.

This explains why an unhealthy diet consisting of a lot of sugar, white flour, colourings and preservatives plays a large part in the development of allergies. Digestive function is disrupted and the immune system weakened by the swamping of the physiological intestinal flora by pathogenic bacteria and fungi. An increased number of pathological bacteria and yeast fungi, especially Candida albicans, produce fusel alcohols and other toxins. The patient is often aware of this in the form of increased accumulation of gas with flatulence, intestinal cramps and irregular bowel movements. What he isn't aware of is that the toxins disrupt the immune system, affect the liver and can impair many other bodily functions through the blood and lymph system.

Problems in the digestive tract

The brain is not spared either: toxins from fungi, bacteria and parasites can lead to inexplicable tiredness, poor concentration and mood swings. And now a vicious circle has developed: the pathological germs and fungi and their toxins encourage the development of food allergies. Food allergies, for their part, irritate the mucous membranes and promote the colonisation of pathogenic germs. This explains why considerable importance is placed on restoring the intestinal flora in allergy therapy.

However most patients know nothing of all this. They come to our practices because they have abdominal pain, cramps, diarrhoea or constipation. If excessive amounts of gas build up, the abdomen becomes distended and those close to the person in question have to bear the unfortunate consequence of large quantities of gas escaping. Before all naturopathic treatment, careful analysis using conventional medical methods with laboratory tests, ultrasound and possibly colonoscopy is essential. It would be inadmissible to treat a patient for food allergies for months, thereby overlooking colon cancer. Generally the patient only comes to us however after he has already consulted a series of conventional medical specialists. Either nothing tangible was found (in which case a psychosomatic disorder is often assumed) or something was found (e.g. chronic inflammation) and symptomatic drug treatment was thought to be sufficient.

Diagnoses such as functional gastrointestinal disorder or irritable bowel syndrome often appear rather awkward descriptions for complaints whose cause has not yet been discovered.

Ten-year-old Niklas came to our practice with his mother because he had suffered persistent abdominal pain and meteorism since the age of 3. One year previously **lactose and fructose intolerance** had been diagnosed by conventional medical methods. The symptoms persisted despite strict abstention. Lactose and fructose intolerance is actually not an allergy. It is a deficiency in the enzymes for breaking down and digesting lactose and fructose. This enzyme deficiency cannot be remedied with bioresonance. Patients often confuse lactose intolerance with allergy to lactalbumin. Lactose intolerance is an inability to digest lactose while lactalbumin allergy is an immunological disorder. Both disorders often occur together. We treated the fungi present in Niklas' intestines and the tested allergies to cows' milk (both lactalbumin and lactose) and fructose. After six treatment sessions the young man was symptom-free and able to eat everything once more.

Problems in the digestive tract

A 40-year-old woman came to us with a violent gastrointestinal complaint. She had **mushy diarrhoea** eight to ten times each day. Part of her stomach had been surgically removed four years previously due to stomach ulcers which had resisted therapy. Despite thorough internal examinations in hospital the cause could not be determined. Shortly afterwards she required surgery for postoperative hernia. In addition to scar interference fields we merely diagnosed wheat allergy. Having removed wheat from her diet the patient was practically symptom-free after a short while and her bowel movements were normal. Four bioresonance therapy sessions were needed to treat the allergy.

A 21-year-old patient complained of digestive problems with abdominal pain, diarrhoea and meteorism which had been ongoing for over six months. A colonoscopy revealed **non-specific colitis**. She refused conventional medication. Kinesiological testing revealed allergies to cows' milk, egg white and citrus fruit as well as intestinal mycosis. After eight sessions with bioresonance therapy her symptoms had largely subsided and her bowel movements were normal.

The non-medical practitioner K.K. reports of a young gynaecologist who worked in a hospital and had suffered from **Crohn's disease** for eight years. She had recurrent severe diarrhoea containing mucous and blood and violent pain in the intestines. The diagnosis of Crohn's disease had been confirmed by means of endoscopy and radiology. At the start of treatment she took cortisone tablets. As a practitioner of conventional medicine, her attitude towards naturotherapy including bioresonance was fairly sceptical. However she continually observed how midwives in the hospital successfully treated pregnant women with homeopathy and acupuncture. At the recommendation of an acquaintance she then went to a naturopathic practice.

Thorough testing with Voll's electroacupuncture revealed cows' milk and wheat allergy as well as Candida mycosis and mercury contamination from amalgam. The allergies to cows' milk and wheat, the intestinal fungi and the disrupted intestinal flora were treated with bioresonance therapy. At the same time amalgam was removed. To regenerate the intestinal flora a preparation with natural intestinal symbionts was prescribed.

The symptoms had already improved markedly after the initial therapy sessions and the cortisone medication could be reduced to a minimum. After 15 treatment sessions the patient was virtually symptom-free and able to eat almost everything once more without

Problems in the digestive tract

any problem.

Fifty-year-old R.R. came to our practice with diarrhoea which had lasted for three weeks. She had suffered from ulcerative colitis in the past yet had been clear of symptoms for 13 years. The patient naturally feared a relapse. Since we had already helped his daughter, he now turned to us for bioresonance treatment. Tests revealed cows' milk allergy and infection with Salmonella typhimurium and Staphylococcus aureus. After avoiding cows' milk temporarily and seven therapy sessions, the patient was largely symptom-free and produced shaped stools once or twice daily.

> Disrupted intestinal flora, fungal infestations and food intolerance are some of the main causes of many chronic gastrointestinal disorders. In many cases, even chronic inflammatory processes such as those found in Crohn's disease and ulcerative colitis can be treated with targeted bioresonance diagnosis and therapy.

Pathogenic influences at the workplace

Occupational diseases

It is difficult if people have to deal with their allergens in their professional life. Here too it is important for the patient to cooperate and bring the substances in question with them to the practice. For our routine test sets are not adequate here. We have already described cases, such as lab technicians, zoo keepers and horse breeders, where animal hair plays a part in the sufferer's working life. But there are also less common animal hair allergens.

A hunter reacted allergically on contact with deer skin. Many animal lovers would have preferred not to treat him at all. Yet we told ourselves too many deer are not good for our forests and treated the environmentally-aware huntsman. A farmer was very happy after we had treated his allergy to cattle hair. Another reacted to chicken feathers. Allergies to goose feathers are not uncommon either. They are often mistaken for allergy to house dust if the patient experiences symptoms tucked up in bed under his down-filled bedding.

But it isn't just animal products which cause problems. Plant products can do so too. What happens when the florist is left gasping for breath on contact with roses, lilac and narcissi? In contrast to the pollen allergy sufferers described earlier, here the plants' fragrance is the culprit. For two years the 50-year-old flower wholesaler R.R. had increasingly been experiencing asthmatic symptoms in his work in the wholesale flower market. In addition to allergies to cows' milk and mould, testing revealed various inhalational allergies to blossoms and foliage he brought with him and also 'sprays' (methoxychlor). He was much better after ten bioresonance therapy sessions and able to continue his work at the wholesale market without becoming short of breath. One year later he was back in touch on account of allergic rhinoconjunctivitis. He brought with him lavender and thyme and also a strip of adhesive tape he had hanging up at his workplace. Many environmental pollutants which are a factor for allergy sufferers can be 'caught' on adhesive tape. After a short time treatment brought relief.

Chemicals at the workplace are a growing problem. A sales assistant became dizzy when unpacking clothing which had been chemically treated. An apprentice painter had

Pathogenic influences at the workplace

coughing fits when he worked with certain paints and varnishes. It's not uncommon for hairdressers to develop eczema from hair dyes and hairsprays. Nurses react to disinfectants and latex gloves.

The Berufsgenossenschaft [statutory accident insurance body] often has to become involved and the person affected risks being declared unfit for work. Retraining costs the taxpayer millions. This is increasingly becoming an economic problem. And, if the patient's occupation was a real 'vocation', the psychological implications may be considerable for the person affected. A joiner had allergic asthma caused by wood dust. He was due to take over the family business. Before deciding to retrain, he wanted to give bioresonance a try. He brought various types of wood dust and the varnishes used in the business with him into the practice. He was able to keep the joinery business – without asthma.

Some more examples in brief (from the book 'Allergie und Schwingung' [Allergy and oscillation]).[14]

An apprentice painter coughed when working with certain varnishes.
A farmer reacted to cattle hair.
A chemical lab technician couldn't tolerate dust from medicines.
A roofer had an allergy to cement and plaster.
A dietician couldn't tolerate lactalbumin.
A hairdresser had eczema from hair dyes.
A businesswoman suffered sneezing fits brought on by her clients' perfume.
A caretaker suffered from a mould allergy.
An engineer had episodes of neurodermatitis from dust at the building site.
A hunter could not tolerate the hair of wild animals.
A cook had an allergy to spices.
A farmer coughed on contact with chicken feathers in the barn.
A butcher had problems working with curing salt.
A scientist couldn't tolerate disinfectants in the laboratory.
A head waiter's eyes streamed when exposed to thick cigarette smoke.
A postman complained of an allergy to printing ink.
A rose seller had an allergy to flowering plants.

---

[14] Dr. med. Jürgen Hennecke, Astro-Spiegel-Verlag, Stolberg, ISBN 3-928830-07-4.

Pathogenic influences at the workplace

A joiner had asthma attacks from wood dust in the workshop.
A clockmaker had an allergy to lubricating oil.
A sales assistant had dizzy spells when unpacking clothing which had been chemically treated.
A wool dealer reacted to wool.
A dentist couldn't tolerate latex gloves.

All were able to continue in their chosen profession after successful bioresonance therapy!

> Work-related allergies cause patients particular difficulty and represent a growing economic problem. Many patients have been saved from ongoing retraining thanks to bioresonance therapy.

Allergological detective work

Uncommon allergens and symptoms

"There is nothing you can't be allergic to." This statement is based upon decades of experience with a wide range of clinical pictures and the most unusual patients. It is essential for the practitioner to determine whether he is dealing with a genuine allergy, a pseudoallergy or an intolerance response. The diagnosis is often the hardest part. How do I find the right substance which is causing the symptoms? Sometimes it is real detective work and the patient's active involvement is essential for this.

A woman came to the practice with allergic rhinoconjunctivitis which had persisted for several months. It was worst in bed in the evening. Obviously all the relevant allergens were tested thoroughly using kinesiology. House dust? Moulds? Bed feathers? Mattress? All negative. Perhaps it was the pillows, the fabric of the bed linen or the detergent? Not that either. Her husband – his after-shave, the smell of his sweat? Negative, thank heavens! But actually it was indirectly connected with the husband: the newspaper! The patient was allergic to printing ink! Whenever the husband read the paper in bed in the evening, the poor woman suffered a sneezing fit.

After a brief ban from the marital bed, her allergy to printing ink and newsprint was treated with bioresonance. Her husband was allowed back into the marital bed – with his newspaper. Conventional medicine would certainly have had even more difficulty reaching a diagnosis.

A student complained of abdominal pain. He noticed the symptoms occurring after he had drunk tea but also after eating vegetable soup and chicken broth. We tested tea, the various types of vegetable and chicken meat. Everything OK. And seasonings or additives? Nothing there either. What was the common denominator? The tap water! This shows how important it is for patients to cooperate and bring the appropriate substances with them from home.

We have since often treated patients who react to their own tap water. It was certainly not an allergy to H_2O but more to chemical substances, which are found dissolved in tap

Allergological detective work

water: chlorine, pesticide and hormone residues, nitrites, nitrates or even heavy metals such as copper and lead from old water pipes.

It is even harder if the reaction occurs, not to individual substances, but to a mixture of different allergens which would not have provoked a reaction separately. An English patient kept complaining of strange muscular twitching. After much searching and testing, the solution to the mystery was found. The culprits were not the milk, coffee or sugar on their own. The allergen was his morning hot coffee with sugar and milk! What went in the Bicom input cup? A glass of hot coffee with sugar and milk! And the muscular twitching disappeared.

He could of course have drunk tea, the keen reader will note. It's not necessary to treat everything; some things you can just do without. This is true in principle. But, to some people, their routines are very important.

With skin rashes, colds, bronchial asthma and enteritis many people immediately think of allergic disorders. But there is also a range of diseases which the therapist trained in conventional medicine does not regard as connected with allergic or allergy-related reactions.

Some patients complain about vague ill health such as tiredness, dizziness and feeling cold. Conventional medical examinations revealed nothing abnormal. Is the patient under a lot of stress? Or are all the symptoms just psychosomatic? Or perhaps there's a hidden food allergy or intolerance? The energetic test makes it all clear.

Did you know that foods which the patient does not tolerate can also cause cardiovascular problems? Inexplicable variations in blood pressure and cardiac irregularity such as frequent premature beats or racing heart may be allergically induced.

It is a little known fact that allergies can also cause bladder symptoms. Patients with irritable bladder suffer from a frequent urge to urinate, pain on passing water and a feeling of pressure in the lower abdomen without yielding a tangible pathological result. Urine samples are completely normal. Lactalbumin was often found to be the responsible allergen in these cases. A milk-free diet with subsequent bioresonance therapy brings relief after a short time. Recurrent urinary infections can also often be

Allergological detective work

attributed to these allergies. The customary antibiotics which are frequently or even permanently prescribed are usually no longer necessary.

Mrs B. P. had suffered from recurrent bladder infections since the age of eighteen. At 46 she was operated on for a wandering right kidney. After this, peritonitis and inflammation of the oral mucous membrane also frequently occurred. The now 62-year-old patient also complained of painful osteoarthritis in the knees and right shoulder and hand which had persisted for three years.

Testing revealed cows' milk allergy and chronic infestation with Chlamydia, amongst other things. Chlamydia is a kind of 'large virus' which, amongst other things, can play a part in respiratory disorders, lower abdominal disorders as well as (when advancing chronically) rheumatoid joint disease.

The scar interference was removed, eliminating organs activated and cows' milk allergy and fungal and Chlamydia infestation treated with bioresonance. After six treatment sessions the patient felt much better. She had had no recurrence of cystitis and even the joint pain was considerably improved. Allergic reactions should also be sought in children who wet the bed at night.

Allergic reaction may play a part in neurological and psychiatric disorders. This includes some forms of tension headaches and migraine. Mood swings and depression, anxiety and panic attacks were a young man's allergic response to eating foods containing hen's eggs. Food allergies are virtually always detected in ADS syndrome which will be examined in more detail later.

Allergic or pseudoallergic reactions even play an important part in some forms of rheumatic disease. In the past a group of types of inexplicable muscular and joint pain, where no antibodies were detected serologically, was often referred to as generalised tendomyopathy. In recent years a more modern term has appeared in reference books and the lay press: fibromyalgia syndrome. The diagnosis is made through a selection of tendon attachment points, which are sensitive to pressure, the so-called trigger points. Unfortunately this diagnosis has not led to any new treatment.

The cause of this widespread disease remains a mystery to conventional medicine

Allergological detective work

although a psychosomatic background is often assumed. Diagnosis is followed by a rather forlorn attempt at treatment with antirheumatic agents, antidepressants and physiotherapy. Nevertheless, it was striking how often the presence of food allergies was observed in this patient group.

The experience of numerous bioresonance therapists leads to the postulation that these foods are not random 'add-ons' but most probably the main cause of the fibromyalgia. Appropriate energetic diagnosis and abstention often resulted in dramatic improvements in the clinical picture. The bioresonance therapist Dr V.M. received a letter from a cured fibromyalgia patient, an extract of which is reproduced here.

"For a number of years (I don't know any more how many it is) I went from one doctor to another as I was suffering from constant pain in every conceivable muscle and always had some block or other in my back or neck. Sometimes these could be remedied with injections (wheals), yet other times this didn't help either. Doctors prescribed remedies for rheumatism but these didn't help and also upset my stomach. I could live with the pain in my back and arms to a certain extent but the pains in my lower legs were a real nuisance and limiting as well (…). By autumn 2002 my life was so restricted that I couldn't clean my house myself as it meant considerable effort. Sleep wasn't refreshing either as I was often awoken by the pain or got up very early in the morning as I couldn't stay lying down.

Some blood counts were taken which were fine according to the doctor. He claimed other people would be glad to have such a good blood count. The constant pain and lack of sleep often made me irritable and my three children and husband suffered because of this (…). The diagnosis was fibromyalgia. The doctor (rheumatologist) explained that the disease was not curable and there was nothing that could be done for it. So there was no need for me to come back again. There was nothing left but to practice gentle sport as movement would enable me to cope better with the stiffness in my muscles… I went to a pain therapist who tried to explain to me that I would be cured if I would look back and reappraise the blows I'd suffered. (…) I then switched to Dr V.M.

I was thoroughly tested (electroacupuncture). (…) that lactic acid can be right-spin or left-spin. This was tested on me and lo and behold, the doctor had found the culprit. We began treatment straight away. After six sessions (bioresonance) I was as good as pain-free.

Allergological detective work

I could look after my home myself once more, carry out my job as clerical worker where before I had sometimes had great difficulty and, slowly but surely, I have begun to do up my home.

But the best thing was New Year's Eve. As I said, I am a cheerful person and have always loved dancing, something I haven't really done for a long time as I'm in such pain shortly afterwards. But last New Year's Eve was different. I was on the dance floor for three hours so that even my friends asked what was up with me, they hardly recognised me…"

There's not much to add to this moving letter. Many therapists have observed that dairy products, and especially lactic acid, obviously play a part in fibromyalgia. One possible explanation could be that the fibromyalgia patient reacts allergically to his body's own lactic acids. Lactic acid is produced in the muscles after severe physical exertion, amongst other things. And what do patients report: muscular pain, intensified following physical exertion. The allergic reaction in the muscle leads to local inflammatory processes with pain.

> Uncommon allergies require meticulous investigation by the therapist with the patient's help. Some symptoms only occur when different substances are combined. In addition to the classic allergic symptoms, many other complaints can be attributed to allergic or intolerance responses.

Own cells under attack

Auto-immune diseases

In the allergic reactions described previously the body produces antibodies or mobilises other defence mechanisms against substances which actually present no threat to it at all. Our immune system was created to identify unwanted intruders and resist or destroy them. Hordes of white blood cells and various groups of antibodies are constantly occupied with eliminating viruses, bacteria, fungi and parasites, thereby preventing the outbreak of disease or starting the process of healing. Yet what threats do pollen, mites or dairy products pose? Why are defence mechanisms launched against these totally harmless substances?

An allergy is an overreaction by an immune system which has been thrown off course. Colds have a biological purpose, namely to eliminate viruses but not, however, as a reaction to birch pollen. Diarrhoea is intended to flush out parasites and not avoid cereal grains. It is even worse if the immune system not only attacks harmless substances from the environment but also the body's own tissue. This is the case with auto-immune diseases. Virtually any tissue and organ can be subject to attack. Two of the most common auto-immune diseases are Hashimoto's disease and Grave's disease. Here auto-antibodies against thyroid tissue are detected in the blood serum. Stimulating antibodies can lead to hyperthyroidism (overactivity). Aggressive antibodies lead to local inflammatory reactions and destroy the thyroid tissue, often ending in hypothyroidism (underactivity). Immune reactions to intestinal epithelial cells lead to Crohn's disease or ulcerative colitis. Antibodies against joint tissue are found in rheumatoid arthritis and Bechterew's disease. Immune reactions to the nerves' myelin sheath, as in multiple sclerosis, occur less frequently.

If antibodies are produced against the body's own DNA, the disease can affect virtually every organ, as is the case with lupus erythematosus. The reason behind the development of auto-immune disorders is still a mystery. It is assumed to be an unfortunate combination of genetic disposition and external factors such as viruses and environmental toxins. A virus which has penetrated the body coincidentally has a very similar surface structure to a thyroid cell, for example. The immune system then

Own cells under attack

produces antibodies to destroy the virus. The thyroid cells are inadvertently destroyed in the process. Conventional medicine does not follow a causal therapeutic approach. Treatment is symptomatic. An underactive thyroid can be treated with replacement therapy and antiphlogistics help against enteritis. In more severe cases, substances which inhibit the immune system such as cortisone or immunosuppressants are used. The high incidence of side-effects from these medicines is well-known.

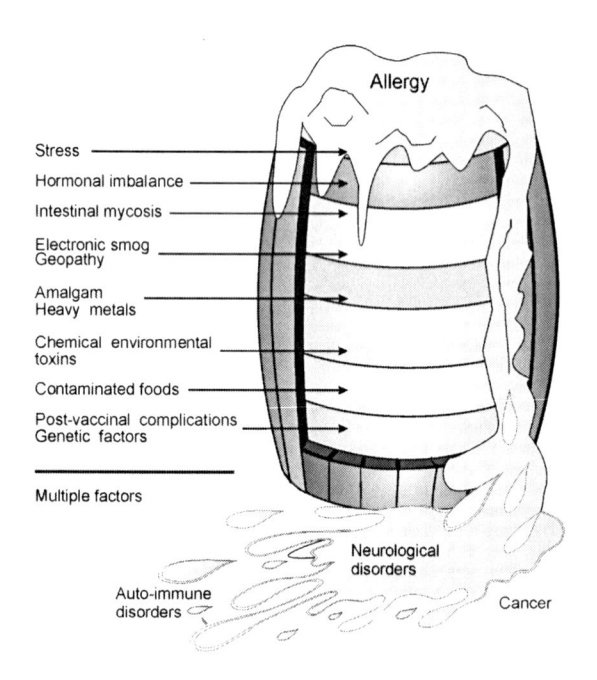

Fig. 21: Chronic diseases are often caused by multiple factors.

Conventional medicine sums up the cause of auto-immune diseases as 'bad luck and the wrong genes.' Holistic therapists don't like to hear the words 'bad luck'. They can't change anything in the genes. They try to track down the adverse factors which are at work here using energetic test methods. Chronic viral and parasitic infections and the adverse effects of inoculations and heavy metals are frequently found with auto-immune diseases. Hidden food allergies, radiation exposure and other energetic blocks also often seem to play a part. It is rare to find just one cause. It is often the interaction between different factors which goad each other on. The body is capable of compensating a large number of negative influences for a long time. But, at some point, the 'barrel' will flood over.

The individual who previously appeared healthy suddenly becomes ill. He had perhaps not noticed minor symptoms in his body or had suppressed them for years. Perhaps he had even provoked his immune system to this through an unhealthy lifestyle. It is even harder to rectify the problem once the damage has been done. Auto-immune disorders are a therapeutic challenge, even for experienced practitioners. The aim of the bioresonance therapist is now to eliminate as many as possible of these adverse factors, to detoxify the body and to stabilise the cells which are still capable of functioning. The disease can often be halted in its advance and some symptoms may improve or disappear. The tissue must be capable of reacting however. If the disease has progressed to the advanced stage, even the bioresonance method has reached its limits. The observation that people with auto-immune diseases are often very sensitive to therapeutic stimuli presents an additional problem. The therapist must proceed with great care and respect in order not to provoke an episode of the disease.

A 56-year-old patient presented at our practice with **hyperthyroid Grave's disease** and chronic sinusitis. She complained of an unpleasant sensation of pressure in her throat and a permanent subjective feeling of unrest. Allopathic medication for hyperactive thyroid had to be discontinued due to intolerance. In addition to hormone imbalance and geopathic stress, kinesiological testing revealed an allergy to cows' milk, house dust and mould. After just three bioresonance therapy sessions the patient already felt subjectively better. The sensation of pressure in her throat had already eased. Since the patient lived some distance away, she was subsequently only treated once or twice each month. In addition to treating the therapy blocks and hormone system, the allergies which had been identified were also treated. Afterwards the patient was practically symptom-free, apart from an occasional slight sensation of pressure in the throat. The results of the lab tests had also improved. For those interested in the technical details: T3 and T4 normal, TSH marginally lower.

The 47-year-old patient M.E. felt completely weary and ill. The conventional medical diagnosis was **euthyroid Hashimoto's thyroiditis**, recurrent arthritis, chronic sinusitis, migraine-type headaches, menopausal symptoms and dyspepsia. The patient changed her sleeping arrangements due to geopathic stress. Intestinal mycoses were rehabilitated and interference from scars following tonsil surgery was eliminated. After just three bioresonance therapy sessions Mrs E. already felt more physically capable, had fewer stomach aches and no more headaches. After a further three treatment sessions the arthritic pain had also disappeared, she felt as fit as a fiddle and was largely symptom-free.

A young patient with **rheumatoid arthritis** came to the non-medical practitioner C. D. for treatment. For over two years she had suffered severe arthritic pain in the joints of the knees, back, hands and feet. She was brought into the practice by her parents as she needed help walking. The slightest movement caused her considerable pain and she was unable to tie her child's shoe laces or open a tin can. The patient had been treated with

Own cells under attack

huge quantities of different medicines which did not help however. Her condition was deteriorating continuously. She refused proposed chemotherapy. She had also suffered from epilepsy since the age of 10.

In addition to treatment with homeopathic remedies and enzymes, bioresonance therapy was also performed. Various programs were used including those for eliminating toxins, releasing blocks and stabilising the kidneys and joints. She already felt much better during the course of the therapy and she took comfort from this. After 16 treatment sessions she was largely symptom-free and it was even possible to reduce her epilepsy medication. Finally she came into the practice wearing smart shoes and announced proudly that she was able to look after her own home and was no longer reliant on outside help. The swelling in her joints had almost completely disappeared. She had a new job as a sales assistant in a shoe shop which she thoroughly enjoyed. She occasionally felt pain in her knees after standing for long periods but her feet were no longer swollen. She was learning to drive and felt tremendously happy.

The non-medical practitioner H.S. reports of a patient who came to his practice having been diagnosed with **multiple sclerosis.** Electroacupuncture testing revealed latent lactalbumin intolerance, chronic infection with herpes virus and post-vaccinal complication from TBE inoculation. At the start of bioresonance therapy the patient complained of feeling extremely tired, of flickering in front of his eyes as well as impaired close vision. This primary immune response disappeared when the treatment was continued carefully.

After a total of 16 treatment sessions the patient was completely symptom-free. A CT scan revealed that the foci detected previously had regressed considerably. The neurologist treating the patient spoke of a 'possible spontaneous recovery' or a potential 'misinterpretation' of the previous pictures. Author's note: 'Spontaneous recoveries' occur with surprising frequency during the course of bioresonance therapy.

> In auto-immune diseases the body produces antibodies against its own tissue. Possible causes of these diseases can be treated effectively with the bioresonance method. Symptoms were observed to improve in thyroiditis as well as in some forms of rheumatic and neurological disease, amongst others.

Latent adverse effects from pathogens

Chronic infectious diseases

Do you know anyone with cold sores? This is an infection with the **herpes simplex virus**. Once the acute symptoms have healed, the virus is not completely eliminated however. It lurks in the nerve cells, lying peacefully dormant and waiting until the host organism's immune system is sufficiently deficient. This can be due to a flu infection, exposure to too much sunshine, sometimes just a negative emotional state such as disgust. Then the virus becomes active once more, reproducing and tormenting its host with a fresh episode of itching and painful sores.

Many people only experience these herpes episodes occasionally and at long intervals. There are patients however who suffer these attacks every few weeks. The eruptions may last for a prolonged period and extend over large areas of skin. Kissing is out of the question and is not the only reason why the sufferer's quality of life is significantly impaired for long periods. We have already been able to help many such patients with three to four bioresonance therapy sessions. These patients then had a break from further cold sore attacks for months and sometimes years.

Treatment takes a two-pronged approach. Programs are applied which, in a non-specific manner, improve the functioning of the immune system and activate defence mechanisms against the virus. Then the virus itself is confronted with its own counter oscillation.

In an acute infection episode virus material can be obtained directly from the content of the cold sore. Appropriate test ampoules are also available however. These ampoules contain either the oscillatory information of the diluted virus material or a potentiated form of administration. A nosode[15] is produced by homeopathic dilution and succussion. This is a medication which, due to its oscillatory properties, is suitable for treating chronic infections of the pathogen in question.

---

[15] Nosodes are sterilised and pyrogen-free remedies, potentiated according to homeopathic principles. The starting material can be micro-organisms (e.g. bacteria), inanimate substances (e.g. contaminants) or healthy or pathogenic organic material (e.g. tissue, secretions).

Latent adverse effects from pathogens

Numerous nosodes have been removed from the market in recent years. The reasons behind this are rather strange. On the one hand it is claimed that the highly diluted nosodes do not contain any molecules from the original substance and are consequently ineffective and, on the other, possible transmission of infection is feared. (Nosode) therapy is still possible with bioresonance and is also completely safe. Nothing is swallowed or injected, simply applied via oscillations.

Other viruses can also lead to chronic infections in the body. The **herpes zoster virus** causes chickenpox or shingles. Even once the scabs have healed, neuralgia often still persists (post zoster neuralgia). Bioresonance therapy can prevent this occurring or alleviate it after the event.

Dr. med F. B. reports of a 76-year-old patient with shingles in the lumbar spine area with sciatica-type radiation into the left leg. The scabs certainly healed following treatment with aciclovir tablets yet the pain persisted. After a further twelve days the pain had spread throughout the whole leg together with a sensation of heat, impaired general state of health and oedema in the instep. The patient was unable to wear proper ladies' shoes and entered the practice limping, supported on her husband's arm. After the first bioresonance treatment session the pain was much better. However the subjective feeling of having a heavy lifeless lump on her leg persisted. After the second bioresonance session the lump feeling had vanished and the patient left the practice with almost a youthful spring in her step. She could fit into her shoes again and went off on a walking holiday to Nepal shortly afterwards.

Epstein Barr virus is increasingly becoming a problem. The acute infection proceeds as **glandular fever (mononucleosis)** with tonsillitis and a high temperature, swollen lymph nodes, rash, arthritic pain, and often hepatitis and enlarged spleen. Unfortunately the manifestations are not always as pronounced as in the textbooks and the disease is often not diagnosed at the acute stage.

Epstein Barr virus is also part of the herpes virus group and tends to remain active long after the acute infection or to be reactivated at 'favourable' opportunities. This often leads to chronic fatigue, reduced vitality, recurrent swelling of the lymph nodes, susceptibility to infection or a tendency to allergy (especially to foodstuffs).

Latent adverse effects from pathogens

14-year-old Michelle had developed glandular fever eight months previously. She subsequently suffered from chronic fatigue and was permanently exhausted. At the same time she developed hypothyroidism (auto-antibodies connected with viral infection). She put on eight kilograms and felt increasingly uncomfortable about herself. Her mother complained that her previously fun-loving daughter had completely changed. Not only was she permanently tired but also moody and aggressive. "She was a different child." Apart from replacement therapy with thyroid medication, conventional medical practitioners were powerless. "You can do what you like; we can't help you", the parents were apparently told by doctors treating their daughter.

In addition to viral infection and the allergies to house dust, animal hair and pollen which had been diagnosed previously, testing revealed chronic allergy to cows' milk. Bioresonance therapy was not easy with Michelle. She had considerable circulatory problems during and after each session so that the therapy programs had to be tailored to her situation and at times reduced. After this she got progressively better. After the 6th therapy session her mother reported that Michelle was no longer as tired and had become more fun-loving. Her behaviour had changed and she was back to her old self again.

Other viruses can also be partly responsible for the occurrence of chronic disease. This includes viruses for cytomegaly, hepatitis, measles and mumps, amongst others. Dr Rummel[16] postulated that chronic viruses play a crucial part in most of the allergic disorders group. He detected raised antibody titres for these viruses in the blood of these patients. Bioresonance therapy via the appropriate virus nosodes is an important step in his treatment approach of 'allergic diathesis' (disposition for allergy).

In **inoculations**, viruses and bacteria in a destroyed or weakened form are injected into the organism. The idea behind the inoculation is to stimulate the immune system to produce antibodies against these germs. In the event of subsequent infection, these can intervene more quickly and prevent or attenuate the disease. One can easily imagine that similar reactions may occur here to those following a genuine infection. Fortunately serious side-effects of inoculations are rare. They must be reported by the doctor and the statistics are monitored. The estimated number of unreported cases is probably much higher.

---

[16] Dr. G. L. Rummel: Bioresonanz, Zukunft und Chance der Medizin [Bioresonance, the future and opportunity for medicine], Verlag Laub GmbH & Co., 2009.

Latent adverse effects from pathogens

Many symptoms are not initially associated with an inoculation which perhaps took place weeks or months before. Children (or adults) will suddenly complain of headaches, abdominal pain, arthritic pain or reduced vitality. Or new allergies occur without any identifiable cause, leading to neurodermatitis, asthma or hyperactivity.

One of the first and most striking examples of post-vaccinal complications in our practice was a doctor's assistant who was 30 at the time. She suddenly succumbed to strange flu-like symptoms: tiredness, headaches and pain in the limbs, yet without a sore throat, cough or high temperature. We first treated her symptomatically with homeopathic remedies, without success. She got progressively worse by the day. The pain in her joints and muscles became so severe that she could scarcely climb the stairs. The blood test which had by now been carried out was largely normal apart from slight eosinophilia. This increase in a subgroup of the white blood cells can indicate worms or allergies. Yet the young woman had never had any allergies before. Finally it occurred to her that she had had a tetanus booster shortly before these vague symptoms appeared. We tested the tetanus ampoule as an adverse influence and immediately treated her with the bioresonance device. Within two days all her symptoms had disappeared.

A 22-year-old student had been suffering from a permanent cold for months. His nose ran almost continuously causing him to consume a huge amount of disposable tissues. Allergy testing for food, house dust and mould allergies did not reveal anything. After a long search the culprit was found: the hepatitis A and B immunisation. He had had this several months earlier in preparation for a trip to Thailand. After two bioresonance sessions to eliminate the vaccine, his nose was clear once more.

We have observed vague abdominal complaints in several young people following hepatitis immunisation. The cervical cancer vaccination for young women is not without its problems either. We have seen headaches, abdominal pain and fatigue and even depressive moods.

Multiple vaccinations are the main factor in small children. The assumption is that the as yet immature immune system is overstretched by being confronted by too many pathogens at once and overreacts. If the child is accordingly disposed, this could trigger allergies and auto-immune disorders or other vague physical or psychological symptoms.

Latent adverse effects from pathogens

Fortunately we have been able to help many patients by 'eliminating' the vaccine with bioresonance, even if the inoculation took place months or years previously. One wonders if all these vaccinations are really absolutely necessary. 30 years ago small children were given 4 inoculations; now 15 are recommended. It might be beneficial to administer individual vaccines at greater intervals. Now mothers bring their children to the practice as a precautionary measure. A bioresonance treatment before the vaccine is administered and prophylactic elimination immediately afterwards can significantly reduce the risk of post-vaccinal complications. This does not affect the protection afforded by the vaccine.

Let's return to infections due to natural causes. In addition to viruses, some species of **bacteria** play an important part. Infection with **Streptococcus** or **Staphylococcus** can lead to angina, sinusitis, bronchitis or dermatitis. We have had patients who were ill with tonsillitis every couple of weeks. Antibiotics were administered continually. The date for the tonsillectomy was already set. One last attempt with bioresonance was successful. In addition to the food allergies present, Streptococcus was repeatedly eliminated. Presumably this reduces the virulence and aggressiveness of the pathogens while at the same time strengthening the immune system's defence against these bacteria. In any event our patients had several months' break before a new infection. Chronic infections with Pneumococcus, Helicobacter and Salmonella have also been treated successfully.

A bacterial disease which recently has occurred with increased frequency and is not always easy to treat is **Borrelia** infection. The pathogens are generally transmitted via ticks as well as other insect bites. The disease develops in three stages. First a red halo, which extends and may migrate (erythema migrans), emerges around the site of the bite. The cutaneous manifestations heal of their own accord after several days. Yet this calm is deceptive. The Borrelia lurk in the organism and may provoke rheumatism-like arthritis many months after the infection (2nd stage). The third stage may manifest itself months or even years after the infection. Neurological symptoms such as headaches, sensory disorders and paralytic symptoms may occur when the nerve cells are affected. Antibiotics afford the greatest help when they are given as soon as possible in the first stage. Bioresonance therapy can have a beneficial effect on the course of the disease at every stage.

Dr B.F. treated a 42-year-old patient who had been suffering pain, swelling and restricted movement in the ankles, knee and wrists since December 1992. Lab tests did not support a rheumatic disorder and fibromyalgia was initially assumed. The patient's

Latent adverse effects from pathogens

hepatic enzyme values were raised and finally a diagnosis was reached on the basis of evidence of antibodies against Borrelia. Several series of antibiotic treatment did not produce any improvement. The doctor first cleansed the colon and treated the patient with phytotherapeutic agents, homeopathic remedies and neural therapy. This alleviated the severe symptoms slightly yet the situation was still on the whole unsatisfactory.

In 1996 Dr B.F. acquired a bioresonance therapy device and began using it straight away with this patient. The patient's quality of life improved considerably as a result. She was able to practice sport once again and cope with her daily routines. Her hepatic enzyme values also improved. However episodes of Borrelia infection in a reduced form flared up with inflammatory joint trouble.

A new attempt with bioresonance was made in 2004. Heavy metals, chemical contamination, mycotoxins, moulds and Borrelia were eliminated with appropriate test ampoules while at the same time the liver was stabilised. This finally resulted in freedom from symptoms. A lengthy process, but one with positive results.

Yeasts such as species of Candida and moulds can also represent chronic burdens for patients. The problem of intestinal mycoses was reported in detail earlier. Moulds like to settle in hollow organs containing air such as the paranasal sinuses and bronchi. They can play a crucial part in chronic sinusitis and bronchial asthma. The toxins produced by fungi such as aflatoxins or fusel alcohols can block metabolic processes.

The role of parasites as the actual cause of many chronic diseases has been discussed in alternative medicine for a number of years. Pioneering work has been produced by the American biologist Hulda Clark. She was even able to treat cancers by consistently eliminating parasites using phytotherapy and zapper technology. The non-medical practitioner Alan Baklayan demonstrated the possibilities of treating parasites with the help of bioresonance and reports on his success in numerous books.

Finally it should be pointed out that not all pathogens which appear as a factor in the energetic test are necessarily responsible for the pathological process. Many viruses, bacteria and parasites populate our bodies without causing any appreciable harm. They then disappear without any special treatment if it is possible to strengthen the organism's overall defence mechanisms.

Latent adverse effects from pathogens

Chronic viral, bacterial, fungal and parasitic infections or those from which the individual did not completely recover can be tracked down and treated using the bioresonance method. It can also have a beneficial effect on health problems following vaccination.

Hidden poison

Chronic toxic contamination

Never over the course of its evolution has the human body had to deal with the level of contamination and environmental toxins it encounters today. In the past there were certainly cases of occupational illness amongst people exposed to heavy metals such as lead, copper, mercury, etc. at work. Modern health and safety legislation has definitely changed things for the better in this respect. Yet, in recent decades, advances in modern chemistry have introduced more and more unnatural products such as pesticides, plastics, colourings, preservatives, to name but a few, into our environment.

The effects are not always felt immediately obvious and are often underestimated. Many types of chronic toxic contamination have no typical symptoms which could indicate the cause. People seek medical help for vague feelings of tiredness, headaches, neurasthenia and other, rather non-specific symptoms of ill health. It is all too easy to claim that stress, which is certainly now also on the increase, is responsible.

Fortunately the body is able to compensate for toxic contamination for a prolonged period as it can identify toxins and segregate and remove them by combining with them biochemically. If this is not sufficient, toxins are also stored temporarily in the fatty and connective tissue to protect the cells of vital organs. Detoxification takes place via the blood and lymph systems and via eliminating organs specifically intended for this purpose. These include the liver and gallbladder system, the kidneys, intestines, lungs and skin. If these systems are overstretched by the quantity or multiplicity of substances requiring detoxification, the symptoms described earlier manifest themselves to an increasing extent.

One of the principal aims of many naturopathic treatment methods is to detoxify and purify the body. This obviously requires an adequate supply of fluids, so patients must drink, drink and drink some more. And preferably large quantities of low-mineral water and not tea, coffee, juice or soft drinks. What do you use to clean a dirty house? Certainly not soft drinks.

Ayurveda, the traditional ancient Indian medicine, recommends drinking large quantities of hot water. The reason for this is that the body does not consume energy heating the cold water up to body temperature and consequently elimination is quicker. This is initially very strange for patients yet they usually accept the idea gratefully and follow the advice.

Another option is to activate the eliminating organs. Naturopathy offers a number of opportunities for doing this. In phytotherapy, teas and medicines containing plant extracts are given to stimulate elimination via the liver, kidneys and lymph glands. Individual and complex homeopathic remedies have a similar effect. Orthomolecular substances such as high doses of vitamins, minerals and amino acids are used as well as seaweed extracts and chelating agents.

These effects can also be achieved with the bioresonance method. Oscillatory information from the eliminating organs and relevant bodily secretions is picked up via electrodes and, once modulated in the bioresonance device, fed back to the body as a specific stimulus. It is also possible to apply stabilising and activating substances and medicines directly. When used on its own, the bioresonance method definitely has an effect. It can also readily be combined with other naturopathic techniques.

As well as these non-specific detoxification measures, the bioresonance method is also able to exert a positive influence on particular toxic substances which harm the organism. Using energetic test methods and appropriate test ampoules it is possible to discover whether the patient is suffering from toxic contamination with chemicals or heavy metals.

Elimination takes place through the bioresonance therapy device. The counter oscillation of the toxin is generated and supplied to the body, in a similar way to that described earlier with allergy therapy. Just like minerals and vitamins, toxic substances are probably unable to penetrate directly through the cell membrane into the interior of the cell. Instead they are first incorporated in a cluster of organised water molecules. The bioresonance oscillation is probably able to disrupt the cluster structure. This achieves two things: the organism is better able to deal with the toxin and can eliminate it from the body more easily. In any case the patient subjectively notices a marked improvement in his symptoms. There are now many examples of successful treatment of acute and chronic toxic contamination with bioresonance.

Non-medical practitioner E. G. reports of a four-year-old boy who returned home from holiday in Turkey seriously ill. He was suffering from frequent nosebleeds, loss of appetite, feeling weak and severe weight loss. He was examined thoroughly in hospital in an attempt to obtain a diagnosis yet no explanation for his condition was found. The boy became increasingly weak and everyone was baffled so that finally his mother consulted a non-medical practitioner. When the boy, hollow-cheeked and his nose bleeding heavily, climbed the stairs to the practice, he was a picture of misery.

In the course of taking the patient's medical history the boy's mother mentioned that they had recently stayed in an excellent, classy new hotel in Turkey. Everything had been fine and the children had spent the whole day in the crystal-clear swimming pool. The older daughter's swimsuit was even completely faded at the end of the holiday.

Mrs E. G. sat up and took notice at this as it could be a sign of the extreme action of chlorine. The non-medical practitioner immediately sent the mother to the nearest chemist to obtain some chlorine. This chlorine was inverted and applied with the bioresonance device. After just two minutes' therapy the boy opened his eyes wide and said: "I'm hungry, Mummy!" His skin became visibly rosy and his whole appearance improved minute by minute. The boy's condition has been stable since then. When the mother subsequently met the therapist, she reported that the boy was as fit as a fiddle, as before.

Progress is not always as swift as in this case of acute chlorine poisoning. Yet the bioresonance method has also proved effective in cases of chronic toxic contamination. A 36-year-old man came to our practice having suffered for years from pain in his upper right abdomen which occurred virtually every time he ate. He had been examined thoroughly using conventional medical methods. For years lab tests had revealed raised hepatic enzyme values so that his GP suspected alcohol abuse. The poor man didn't touch a drop of alcohol however, as he convincingly assured us. Thorough kinesiological testing revealed toxic contamination with methoxychlor and lindane. The patient then reported that he had worked for years in horticulture and these substances were used as pesticides for Christmas trees and other plants. This was a long time ago however and he now worked as a dog trainer. We activated liver detoxification with bioresonance and eliminated the two toxic substances. After six treatment sessions the pain after eating had disappeared and his hepatic enzyme values had improved. For those interested in the technical details: the gamma GT level fell from 315 to 120 and even the cholesterol level improved from 254 to 207!

It is not uncommon for toxic contamination to test positive as the cause of patients' disorders. Chronic contamination with formaldehyde and wood preservatives was frequently found. Xyladecor stain and Xylamon woodworm treatment were used in the sixties and seventies to preserve wooden ceilings and garden fences. After testing, patients often report that they have lived for years in a home with wooden floors or wooden ceilings or had varnished these themselves.

Astonishingly, symptoms which had persisted for years improved after being eliminated with bioresonance although there was currently no contact with the toxic substances in question. Toxic contamination from heavy metals also quite often tests positive, for example lead from old water pipes or aluminium after using old saucepans for years.

The most frequently tested heavy metal is mercury. As this is the main constituent of amalgam fillings in teeth, court cases brought against amalgam manufacturers by injured patients have been running for years. Despite numerous expert reports the courts have been unable to reach a conclusive decision. The use of amalgam fillings has been prohibited in pregnant women and children, however. Is mercury harmless then for everyone else?

The experiences of many naturopathic therapists give a clear message. After careful removal and replacement of amalgam by a dentist followed by subsequent detoxification, the symptoms of many chronically ill patients improved where conventional medical treatment had been unable to help.

Dr M. C. reports of a patient in her late 20s who had been suffering from tinnitus in both ears for 10 years and consequently was severely depressed to the point of contemplating suicide. After therapy for food allergies and amalgam detoxification, the tinnitus disappeared completely, a fact confirmed by the ENT specialist.

Hidden poison

A 32-year-old woman came for removal and replacement of amalgam since she was not happy with her weight. After three therapy sessions she had already lost four kilos. At the end of the treatment she reported the symptoms which had improved as a result: weariness, lack of concentration, neurasthenia, irritability, headaches, pain in the back of the neck, oedema in the eyelid, diarrhoea, rashes, coating on the tongue and dry mouth!

> Acute and chronic poisoning by heavy metals and chemicals can be treated by stimulating the eliminating organs energetically and specific biophysical detoxification therapy. Patients' symptoms usually improve rapidly.

The sensitive nervous system

Neurological disorders

The nervous system contains our organism's most highly specialised cells. It is an effective high-speed communication system reaching right into our body's many different organ areas with their individual specialist roles.

A distinction is made between the central nervous system with the brain and spinal canal and the peripheral nervous system with its sensory, motor and vegetative nerve fibres branching into the furthest tissue and organ cells. It not only provides and processes all sensations but also produces all emotional and physical impulses including the fine motor system of our limbs. Consequently the system is highly susceptible to interference.

Pathological changes may affect either the cell itself, the myelin sheath wrapped around the nerve trunk or the synapses which maintain communication between the nerve cells through specific mediators.

The symptoms of disorders of the nervous system range from pain such as neuralgia and neuropathy, disorders affecting sensation and perception, vegetative dysfunction, motor disturbance such as tremors and paralysis to psychological conditions such as anxiety, depression, loss of concentration and hyperactivity. The most common causes of neurological disorders are toxic contamination with heavy metals or neurotoxic chemicals (e.g. insecticides), neurotropic viruses (e.g. herpes virus) or bacteria (e.g. Borrelia), allergic or autoimmune processes (e.g. through inoculations) and psychological causes. Bioresonance has no effect on the latter yet considerable success with neurological disorders has already been recorded by treating the other detrimental factors.

Examples of successful bioresonance treatment for migraine and tension headaches, postherpetic neuralgia, nerve irritation in orthopaedic syndromes, multiple sclerosis and many other conditions have already been presented in the relevant chapters of this book.

In some disorders the connection between toxins, pathogens and symptoms is well-known and accepted in conventional medicine. However, these detrimental influences cannot always be detected by lab tests and imaging processes. The treatment options available in conventional medicine are also often very limited and associated with serious side-effects.

Energetic testing is far more sensitive for this purpose as it can detect, not only the material presence of these factors, but even the information they contain. And it is possible to measure the energy levels of this information if physical contact took place some time in the past. And even more interesting: if this disease-inducing information is deleted with bioresonance, the symptoms improve markedly in most cases.

A 35-year-old man came to the practice of non-medical practitioner A. K. with a **tremor** in his left hand, **migraine attacks** and **lapses of memory**. A year previously he had been given a tetanus and hepatitis B inoculation and anti-malarial drugs as he was traveling abroad in his job. The migraine set in four weeks after the inoculation; the tremor developed within four to five months. Twelve bioresonance treatment sessions were necessary in which the vaccines were eliminated, amongst other things. After this the migraine and lapses of memory were gone; the tremor had also virtually disappeared. It merely reoccurred briefly in a mild form in stressful situations.

An eighteen-month-old child with **developmental disorders** who **cried continuously** was brought to the same practice. He was not yet able to sit unaided or crawl and was not really interacting with his environment. The mother explained that her child had had a hexavalent vaccine at the age of eight weeks and had reacted with a high temperature and spasms. He no longer slept through the night after this. The child woke with a start, cried and was almost impossible to pacify. Doctors told the mother her child had autistic traits. Post-vaccinal complications were the main cause of this too.

After six bioresonance therapy sessions there was a dramatic change in the child. He began to seek eye contact and was more aware of his surroundings. After a further six therapy sessions the child was able to sit unaided. In addition to the post-vaccinal complications, food intolerance was also treated. Only now did the occupational therapy, which the child had already been receiving for over a year, work. One year later the child was able to walk and started to say simple words.

The sensitive nervous system

The Egyptian doctor Dr H. M. reported at the 2004 Bioresonance Congress on the successful treatment of children with **cerebral palsy** using bioresonance combined with physical therapy. Cerebral palsy is a dysfunction of the first motor neuron, in other words the nerve cell which provides the impulse to move the muscles.

Cerebral palsy is the most well-known neuromuscular disorder in children. It may be congenital or develop in the first five years of life. It is linked with disturbance to the motor system and posture. The cause may be lack of oxygen, bleeding, infection and genetic abnormalities.

Eleven-year-old M. T. had cerebral palsy of unknown origin. Despite physical therapy the spasticity of the upper and lower limbs increased. His neck reflexes were completely absent and he was unable to bend his hips or keep them firm or maintain the balance in his trunk. He just lay in bed, without moving or reacting and was incapable of communicating.

The bioresonance method was then used in addition to physical therapy. After four months he was able to sit with his legs crossed at the knees and back supported. First the deformities in the elbows disappeared, then after six months those in the knees. Now he could control his head and sit on a chair. He responded to acoustic and visual stimuli. After eight months he was able to sit on a ball and maintain his balance. His understanding grew and he recognised his parents. He drew attention to himself through emotional responses like crying so that his parents would place him in front of the TV. For years he had lain unnoticed wrapped up in his own world. Now he sat in front of the TV and took pleasure from the children making music and singing.

A 49-year-old man, W. A., suffered from **severe depression** with lack of vitality, exhaustion and loss of concentration. The first symptoms of exhaustion had appeared back in 1982. At the same time he noticed itchy blotches on his skin, pain in the knees, back and back of the neck as well as tingling in the hands. Four years later depression, decrease in vitality, problems concentrating and impaired vision were added to these symptoms. He subsequently developed a sore throat, intra-ocular pressure and mild paralysis in the left side of the face.

Two weeks' thorough investigation in the state mental hospital failed to yield any results.

In 1988 he was back in hospital with severe chest pains. A heart attack was ruled out. One year later an attempt was made to place a 'protective shield' beneath his amalgam fillings as he was suffering from toothache.

Eight week's treatment in a psychosomatic clinic restored his health somewhat. On his return he developed severe headaches after having a new amalgam filling which only disappeared after the filling was removed. He was given another full internal check and the symptoms were declared to be a psychosomatic disorder.

When he came to Dr B. B. for treatment, he had considerable physical and mental problems once more. It emerged from taking the patient's medical history that many years previously when building his house he had worked with a lot of wood preservatives. A lab test was performed which showed raised PCB (polychlorinated biphenyl) levels in his blood. His wife and son were also contaminated with PCBs. There was no option for the family but to leave the house temporarily and move in with the father-in-law. In addition to contamination with wood preservatives and amalgam, energetic testing also revealed cows' milk intolerance. A dentist removed and replaced the amalgam fillings and detoxified the mercury deposits, while the patient maintained a milk-free diet as instructed.

At the same time the contamination with wood preservative was treated with bioresonance. The patient brought various fabric fibres and painted pieces of wood from the house with him for this. The depression completely disappeared during this treatment. After treating the milk allergy all his other symptoms, such as joint pain, intra-ocular pressure and chest pain, also vanished. He felt like a new person. His mental state, which had got out of control, had returned to normal and was stable once more. The family never moved back into the house again.

Physical and psychological complaints due to toxic substances in buildings have now entered the literature as 'sick building syndrome'. To sum up, chronic poisoning from environmental toxins and heavy metals and also food intolerance should always be considered in the case of vague psychological symptoms such as depression, loss of concentration, anxiety and panic attacks. Bioresonance therapy is generally helpful for these patients. There is not yet sufficient experience available in the case of endogenous depression and psychoses.

The sensitive nervous system

In this connection we also want to mention at this point the problem of a condition which is becoming an increasing challenge in our society and which is affecting a growing number of children (and adults): **attention deficit disorder (ADD)** with or without hyperactivity **(ADHD)**. In the past these children were described in belittling tones as dreamers or fidgets. But those affected, and even more so, parents and teachers do not find it so humorous. Depending on the severity, the conventional medical approach is to use psychosocial intervention or medication. There is not yet sufficient information available on the side-effects of long-term use of this medication.

Energetic test methods detect one or (often) more of the detrimental factors listed here in these patients: allergies or intolerance to milk, wheat, sugar, colourings and preservatives as well as foods containing phosphate, infestation with Candida or herpes virus, toxic contamination with heavy metals or chemicals, post-vaccinal complications or problems caused by medication. It can be helpful to take a thorough medical history of the patient.

Parents or teachers frequently report that, after eating sweets (sugar and colourings!), the child is jumping over tables and benches. If these are eliminated from the child's diet, it is well behaved and attentive. We made the interesting discovery that substances and medication which the mother took, or was prescribed, during pregnancy tested positive as detrimental factors in the child in energetic testing (!).

After treating and eliminating these substances from the child using bioresonance, symptoms generally improve markedly. In one case the mother had been given diazepam (a tranquilizer) during pregnancy, to calm her, due to premature labour pains. After appropriate elimination with bioresonance, ADD medication could be discontinued.

The child is possibly suffering continuously from withdrawal symptoms (see also 'Addictions' chapter). In another case the mother had smoked hashish during pregnancy. We had her bring the substance with her and treated the child with it. Successfully!

The non-medical practitioner A. K. reported of a five-year–old boy with severe ADD syndrome. While the mother explained why she had come, the boy clambered around on the treatment couch in the consulting room, touched everything on the desk, talking all the while. Finally he did somersaults on the carpet. As you can imagine, energetic testing

The sensitive nervous system

required considerable effort and patience on the part of the therapist.

Post-vaccinal complications and food allergies were diagnosed. The practice staff complained after the treatment session that the boy had been impossible. He had fidgeted, spat and uttered words which cannot be repeated here due to child protection legislation. His symptoms worsened after the first treatment session and the mother wondered whether she should continue. After a proper discussion with her and explaining about possible initial exacerbation, she came to a second therapy session. The boy was now much more affable.

After six therapy sessions the post-vaccinal complications had been remedied so that the food intolerance could be treated. After this the boy was a different person. There were no more problems at nursery school and peace was restored in the family.

> Neurological disorders can frequently be attributed to the chronic influence of environmental toxins and viruses. Symptoms usually improve dramatically after appropriate elimination. There are also positive reports of treatment of ADD and ADHD.

Pain warning signs

Pain syndromes

Pain is a nature's clever way of signalling to us that something is wrong with our body. Specific pain receptors pass this information in a fraction of a second via nerve fibres to our brain where it is processed and reaches our consciousness. Perception of the intensity of the pain depends largely upon cultural and individual circumstances. Pain receptors are most often stimulated by injury or inflammatory processes.

In earlier times this was a signal for people to stay calm, get into a position which did not aggravate the pain and give the body the opportunity to heal. Today pain is a signal for people to reach for a tablet or run to the doctor.

Pain research has made considerable progress in recent years. The term pain memory is used especially in connection with chronic pain. We now know exactly how pain arises and have developed various strategies for influencing the various stages by pharmacological means. Treatment strategies which do not involve medication have also been known for a long time: use of heat and cold, cupping and massage, stimulation current and magnetic fields, lasers and X rays are all part of the pain therapist's arsenal. The pain-relieving action of acupuncture has already been the subject of scientific research. Assuming that a biophysical field change precedes all biochemical metabolic processes in the body, this ought also to apply to pain. In other words: bioresonance should, in theory, also work for pain and, in practice, it actually does.

The experience of thousands of patients proves the ability of bioresonance to relieve pain. "Pain is tissue's cry for flowing energy," (quote from Dr Voll). The electrode in the resonance device 'hears' this cry and sets blocked energy moving again. In the case of acute pain, its occurrence can be directly influenced by placing the electrodes in a specific position and by selecting certain program parameters. In the case of chronic pain, detrimental factors such as therapy blocks, allergic conditions and toxic contamination and viral and parasitic infestation are specifically sought to treat these as causal influences where possible. Let's look at pain patients from **head to foot.**

Pain warning signs

Headaches are one of the most common forms of pain in general medical practice. Apart from some more unusual cases such as tumours or neurological disorders, most patients suffer from various forms of tension headache or migraine.

12-year-old Benedikt had suffered **migraine-type headaches** since starting school. Recently the attacks had been occurring weekly with pain alternating between the forehead and temples, linked with severe nausea. His parents did not want to give him strong painkillers and first tried homeopathic remedies, unfortunately without much success. He tested positive for cows' milk allergy and contamination with the wood preservative Xyladecor. He had slept in a room with an old wooden ceiling for years. After cutting milk out of his diet temporarily, the allergy was treated with bioresonance and the wood preservative eliminated. The young man was already much better after just five therapy sessions; the headaches occurred only very occasionally in a milder form, the nausea had disappeared and he was able to sleep better.

The dentist Dr med. dent. H. V. reports of a 63-year-old patient with pain from the onset of **osteoarthritis in the right temporomandibular joint**. She had already been wearing a dental splint for three years. The pain arose on opening the mouth. In addition, terminal cracking sounds and a slight deviation to the right of the lower jaw at the end of the mouth were observed. The programs for correcting temporomandibular and hyoid bone blocks were conducted in a total of eight weekly treatment sessions. After this, the patient was in no pain and no longer needed to wear the splint either.

A 58-year-old patient had been suffering for over 30 years from **cervical spine syndrome**. She had already consulted over 20 health practitioners but with only very moderate success. After just two bioresonance therapy sessions she felt much better. She had monthly treatment. She no longer needed chemical pain killers. Around 70% improvement. Patient's comment: "Now I have my life back".

In conventional pain therapy even a subjective 50% pain alleviation is regarded as successful treatment.

A 63-year old Greek man complained about pain in his right **shoulder blade** and right buttock. This had begun four years previously following a stroke resulting in paralysis of the right side of the body. Fortunately the paralysis had completely receded but not the pain however. He had consulted three orthopaedic surgeons, a pain therapist, several physiotherapists and an acupuncturist – all without success. We treated intestinal mycosis, neutralised radiation exposure, eliminated interference from the stroke scars in his head and applied a pain program to the affected parts of the body. All the pain had disappeared after three bioresonance therapy sessions!

Dr med. P.-G. V. treated a 48-year-old patient with **chronic pain following a comminuted fracture of the elbow**. She had suffered the injury eleven years previously and at that time had to have surgical osteosynthesis. Since then she had suffered extreme pain which even antirheumatic agents could barely control. After just three sessions of bioresonance pain therapy on consecutive days the patient was symptom-free. Symptoms reappeared once more after a few weeks. The above-mentioned therapy was repeated three times. After this, the symptoms disappeared again and the patient remained symptom-free for about five months. When the pain recurred the therapy was repeated again and, since then, the patient has now been able to play tennis once more without pain.

The same doctor treated a 68-year-old patient with **recurrent lumbago** following two operations on her intervertebral discs. She was unable to carry anything heavy without immediately incurring symptoms. Orthopaedic treatment had so far proved unsuccessful. An attempt to treat her condition with homeopathic remedies brought only short-term relief. Eight therapy sessions were carried out, twice a week. A special roller electrode was used as well as programs for eliminating scar interference, slipped disc and pain in the lumbar spine. The patient was symptom-free after four weeks. It was possible to feel the extent to which the back muscles had relaxed. The patient was now able to lift even very heavy cases and her movements were not restricted.

The Congress paper by the Turkish doctor Ö. K., who works as a neurosurgeon both in her own practice and in the city hospital in Istanbul was remarkable. She summarised her experience: "Since using the bioresonance method the number of operations on **slipped discs** has fallen considerably. You could say that, unaware of the bioresonance method, my team and I reached for the scalpel much too often and too prematurely in the past. Over a twelve month period 124 patients with lumbar (53) and cervical (71) slipped discs (hernias) were treated exclusively with bioresonance. The diagnosis of 2nd or 3rd degree slipped disc, in some cases with neurological deficit, was established in all the patients by

Pain warning signs

means of imaging techniques e.g. MRI.

The patients were all treated exhaustively with conventional medical methods and were referred for surgery by colleagues. All patients responded well to bioresonance treatment. On average, 12 sessions per patient were required. MRI images were then prepared to check the patients' condition. 2nd degree slipped disc could no longer be detected radiologically, 3rd degree hernias had receded significantly."

Two case studies will demonstrate the effect of the neurosurgeon's treatment. The 77-year-old patient P. S. came to the practice completely exhausted because she had hardly slept for three weeks due to severe pain in the lumbar region and in the legs. The orthopaedic surgeon treating her had prescribed physical therapy which increased the pain. She had osteoporotic compression fractures and consequent severe scoliosis. Her spine was also worn with herniated discs at several levels. The pain had already receded markedly after the first therapy session alone. After five sessions she was completely pain-free.

The 68-year-old patient F. A. had paralysis of the feet (foot drop), for two years on the left side and six months on the right side. The patient had already been urged two years before to have surgery as a matter of priority. From a conventional medical viewpoint it was an absolute neurosurgical emergency. However, the patient refused surgery despite her condition deteriorating. At the start of the bioresonance treatment the doctor did not hold out much hope for the patient or herself due to the severity of the situation. Treatment lasted four months in all and resulted in 100% remission.

54-year-old I. S. had had a left **hip endoprosthesis** fitted two years previously. Since then she could no longer put weight on her leg properly. She complained of wandering pain on the outside of the left thigh and the back of the left buttock. Dr med. W.-D. K. administered eight bioresonance therapy sessions at three day intervals. On completion of the treatment the patient could once again walk without crutches and put weight on the foot on the painful side without any problems.

A 63-year-old patient who had suffered **arthritis of the knee** for many years had severe problems walking and standing. She travelled some distance for ten day's treatment with Dr med. G.-P. V. The patient felt a marked improvement after just three bioresonance treatments. She could walk much better and further than before. At the end of the treatment she was completely symptom-free and able to resume her job as a sales assistant. A success which orthopaedic surgeons had previously been unable to achieve with her.

40-year-old I. M. had a motorbike accident as a young man tearing the ligament of his **left ankle**. Since then he complained of constant pain in his foot, especially after putting weight on it. A major disadvantage for a keen tango instructor. He also had chronic tension in the cervical spine area following a whiplash injury. After five bioresonance therapy sessions he was symptom-free and now able to continue his passion for dancing.

It is not only pain from orthopaedic conditions which can be treated successfully with bioresonance. This method can also address neuralgia and pain in the abdomen and lower abdomen.

> Acute and chronic pain in all parts of the body can be quickly relieved in most cases.

Degenerated cell growth

Malignant diseases

Scarcely any diagnosis evokes as much anxiety and emotion as that of cancer. In many people the word alone triggers a succession of thoughts and feelings including panic, suppression and confrontation with their own inevitable death (at some future point). Yet, in the initial stages, cancer is quite curable and, even in the advanced stages of the disease, a great deal can be done to improve the quality and extend the life of most patients. On receiving this diagnosis only a few people opt purely for alternative medicine. Most patients avail themselves of the treatments offered by conventional medicine, namely surgery and, if necessary or possible, chemotherapy and/or radiotherapy.

Cancer patients will clutch at any straw offered and increasingly are looking for supportive alternative therapies in addition to conventional treatment. They hope to reduce the side effects of conventional treatment, improve their quality of life, support their body's immune system and, where possible, also directly inhibit the tumour. The market in alternative methods of treating cancer is now quite extensive and includes mistletoe extracts, enzymes, high doses of vitamins and minerals, probiotic agents, homeopathic remedies, hyperthermia, anti-cancer diets and many others.

Most of these methods are still derided by conventional medicine. Serious positive studies already exist for some methods (e.g. mistletoe therapy), while evidence of the effectiveness of others is not yet available. But many conventional medical statistics are not completely reliable either, if patients use alternative therapies, perhaps without their attending doctor or the 'statistician' knowing. If several treatment strategies were used, no-one can say afterwards what really helped the patient. It might even have been the combination of different methods which led to the success of the treatment. Ultimately it is all the same to the patient.

The bioresonance method is also used with cancer patients but almost always in combination with other conventional and alternative methods. There are a number of reports by patients and therapists of successful treatment but it is not yet possible to

Degenerated cell growth

produce a reliable set of statistics (as with allergy therapy).

What strategy should bioresonance therapists pursue? As with other chronic disorders, with cancer patients they will also want to eliminate therapy blocks, stimulate detoxification, stabilise the immune system, improve metabolism and vitality and, if possible, slow down tumour growth directly. Ideally they should start with the cause. But what does cause cancer? The factors triggering a number of types of cancer are well-known, such as toxins (e.g. cigarette smoke), chemicals, medicines, viruses, radiation, etc. Alternative medicine has added to this a few 'suspected' causes such as parasites, foods, etc. The influence of the individual's mental state is also continually debated.

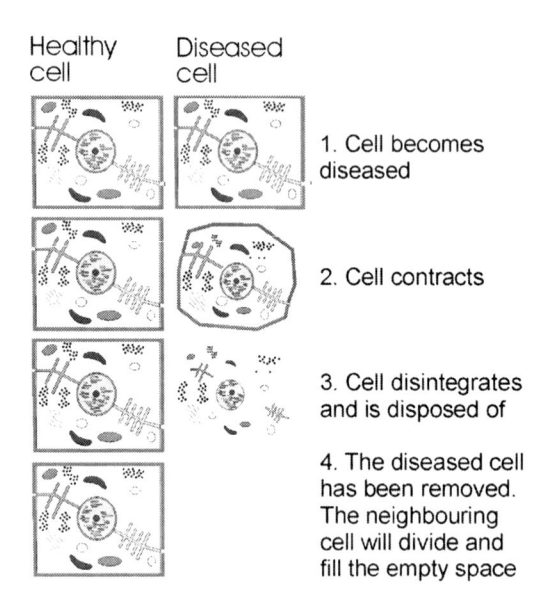

Fig. 22: Apoptosis: programmed death of diseased and old cells.

1. Cell becomes diseased
2. Cell contracts
3. Cell disintegrates and is disposed of
4. The diseased cell has been removed. The neighbouring cell will divide and fill the empty space

So cancer seems to represent the immune system's capitulation before a seemingly insurmountable mountain of 'rubbish' in the organism; the final stage of a prolonged negative process evolving over many years with the collapse of the body's ability to heal itself. One of the most interesting theories in recent years for the development of cancer is linked to the phenomenon of apoptosis, or voluntary cell death.

Our bodies' cells all have a limited life and are continually being replaced. Red blood corpuscles, for example, live for around 100 days, i.e. new blood flows through our arteries after 3.5 months. All the bodies' cells are replaced once every couple of months. The person you see in the mirror today is not the same one you looked at six months ago, materially speaking, even if you cannot tell the difference. For every new cell created one old one must die so that you maintain the same body size and shape. Otherwise your body would keep growing continuously.

The organism has developed a finely tuned system to bring about this controlled cell death. Scientists have discovered that all healthy cells have a suicide gene (p53 gene)

Degenerated cell growth

which, when activated, causes the aged cell to die. The neighbouring cells in the cell group play a crucial role in this. They produce chemical mediators (and biophotons?) which bring about cell death at the right moment. But what happens when this mechanism is no longer functioning properly? The cells reproduce without the old cells being removed from the cell group, leading to tumour growth. Tumour cells are usually more primitive cells than mature body cells. They are identified as alien by the immune system and quickly destroyed before they can wreak too much havoc.

Scientists assume that thousands of tumour cells are produced each day in our bodies which are then identified and destroyed by our immune system. But what happens if the immune system no longer performs this task properly?

A series of test and therapy ampoules has been developed for bioresonance whose oscillatory information is intended to act specifically on these mechanisms. The tissue surrounding the tumour is stimulated to promote apoptosis or the death of the tumour cells! The immune system is stabilised with other ampoules. Thorough training and experience with the bioresonance method is required to work with these highly effective ampoules. The therapist uses general stabilising therapy measures in addition to this specific tumour therapy. These include neutralising the geopathic stress which almost inevitably exists, eliminating interference from surgical scars, eliminating toxins and stabilising the immune system.

The Turkish doctor, Dr Ö. K. treated a 22-year-old patient who presented with symptoms of fatigue and vague syncopes (fainting fits). A **brain stem glioma** was diagnosed using magnetic resonance imaging. The neurosurgeon who was called in told the patient that the only treatment for this type of tumour was regular MRI scans. Other treatments were not effective. At this Dr. Ö. K. treated the patient with bioresonance. Amongst other things, energetic testing revealed a reovirus infection, heavy metal contamination with mercury, palladium and nickel and a cows' milk allergy.

A milk-free diet was prescribed, the viruses and heavy metals were eliminated and the patient was treated with the special tumour test set ampoules. After seven months, energetic testing produced negative results and an MRI scan was performed. There was no longer any sign of a tumour! The doctor treated five other tumour patients. These

Degenerated cell growth

had been operated on and had had chemotherapy. Bioresonance therapy was used afterwards. Programs for toxin elimination together with supportive and fortifying therapies were used. Compared with other patients who were not treated with bioresonance, these patients were in a much better state.

> Many cancer patients are looking for additional naturopathic therapies alongside conventional methods of treatment. The immune system can be supported and therapy blocks eliminated with biophysical methods. Apoptosis and consequently tumour growth may possibly also be influenced.

When enjoyment becomes an addiction

Dependency symptoms

What is the connection between addiction and allergy? Since the 1970s '**clinical ecology**'[17] has supported the theory that addictive behaviour is based on an intolerance reaction, in other words, a special form of 'allergy' to a particular substance. A foodstuff acting 'allergically' can therefore trigger two conflicting behaviour patterns in the affected person.

The first pattern is **rejection**. The food is instinctively avoided because the body senses that it harms it. If we diagnose a milk allergy in a patient, for example, they will often report that, right from childhood, they never liked milk. Their parents forced them to drink milk however because it was 'so healthy'. The parents certainly acted in good faith and could not know that they were laying the foundation for the occurrence of other allergies or other diseases in their child.

The second behaviour pattern is **craving** for the food which acts 'allergically'. It is often consumed in large quantities and, if it is not available, proper withdrawal symptoms may appear or the person will at least feel unwell or manifest a reduced general state of health. What could be the reason for this unnatural behaviour? The body is possibly completely unable to process this substance which it cannot tolerate and is unable to integrate it usefully in its metabolism. This leads to an apparent deficiency in this substance which can only apparently be rectified by increased consumption. Clinical ecologists believe this may be one of the main causes of addictive behaviour.

I'm sure you have heard comments like: "I need a coffee to wake up in the morning", "I need my glass of milk or I'm no fun", "I need my chocolate or I'm in a bad mood", "I need sugar or I have no energy", "I need a cigarette…, I need my glass of beer…, I need…, I need… etc." Isn't this a case of addictive behaviour due to an allergic reaction? I'm sure you know people who crave something sweet and, when they have eaten it, feel really

---

[17] Clinical ecology deals with irritants occurring in the environment, together with the associated symptoms of allergies, intolerances, intoxications, etc. as well as their treatment.

When enjoyment becomes addiction

unwell? And yet they can't give it up. And if that isn't an addiction!

In this case the allergen does not produce symptoms in the skin, respiratory tract or the intestines but evidently in the brain. The symptoms are not a rash or mucous congestion but psychological changes. These food allergens play a large part in ADD syndrome.

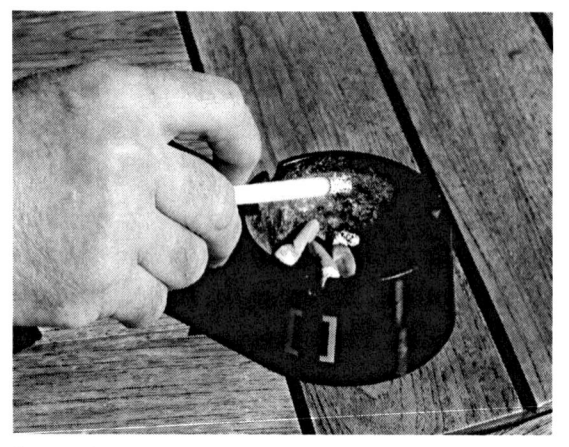

Fig 23: An increasing number of patients want to give up smoking.

If the relevant substances are treated with the techniques of bioresonance allergy therapy, patients generally observe that they can suddenly manage well without this substance. They no longer experience a craving, feel freer and no longer have withdrawal symptoms such as agitation, neurasthenia and sleeping disorders, etc.

The fact that smoking damages health does not need further explanation here. You can now read examples on every cigarette packet. Despite all the public information campaigns, over 50% of all young people today still start smoking and subsequently over 80% of them want to give up again. That is easier said than done, however. Many have already tried once or more times. They were often unsuccessful or started smoking again having given up for a certain period, sometimes even quite a long break.

Smoking is increasingly a drain on the wallet so that patients are prepared to invest some of this money in actually quitting the habit. Various methods are available on the market. There are nicotine chewing gums and nicotine patches where the addictive substance is supplied to the body in a different form to reduce withdrawal symptoms. By slowly reducing the dose the body is weaned off the habit. Psychopharmaceuticals are also deployed which are designed to work directly on the addiction centres in the brain; not without side-effects, however. Acupuncture is also reported to be successful. Acupuncture points on the body or ears are stimulated with needles or laser beams and these correct the autonomic nervous system and check the addictive behaviour.

When enjoyment becomes addiction

Bioresonance smoking cessation is based on the aforementioned theory that addiction and allergy operate by similar mechanisms. The main part of the therapy consists of 'allergy treatment for cigarettes'. This is performed using the same counter oscillation programs which are also used to eliminate toxins. The body is encouraged to stop reacting to this substance in an excessive and uncontrolled manner and at the same time to eliminate it, in other words, rid the organism of it. To accompany this, basic therapy and programs for the lungs, breathing, metabolism and general detoxification are also used. The motivation to want to quit has to come from the patients themselves.

Non-medical practitioner B. K. reports of a patient who successfully completed smoking cessation therapy in her practice and then worked on her son-in-law: "You're going to quit now too!" Together with her (non-smoking) daughter she bullied the young man and dragged him into the practice. He stood there complaining: "What a load of rubbish! I don't even want to give up. What's the point?" But, to keep everyone quiet, he went along with it - he was outnumbered after all! He was very sceptical about bioresonance therapy yet agreed to undergo the full procedure for standard smoking cessation therapy. And guess what; from that moment on he hasn't smoked a single cigarette. He simply no longer craved a smoke and, one year later, nothing had changed.

In July 2005 an article appeared in the Sunday Telegraph in which a British journalist reported on bioresonance smoking cessation therapy: "When the electrode was placed on my forehead, I began thinking about all my attempts to stop smoking and came to the conclusion that this was probably the most ridiculous. But it worked!" In the light of this article the television broadcaster Channel 4 invited the journalist and the bioresonance therapist onto a chat show. The TV programme led to the therapist's practice being inundated with enquiries so that, in the end, she even had to take up the professional help of a call centre to manage the incoming calls.

If bioresonance works so well with nicotine addiction, how good is it at treating other addictions such as alcohol and drugs, etc? Here too there are promising beginnings. A clinic in Poland is using bioresonance to treat alcoholics and drug addicts. There are reports of success here too. However, with serious clinical pictures such as these, bioresonance can only be one part of a comprehensive treatment plan in which the psychological and social care of the patient is extremely important.

When enjoyment becomes addiction

> Clinical ecology describes addiction as a special form of allergic reaction. This explains how bioresonance has been successful in addiction therapy. Many smokers have been freed from their dependency.

Bioresonance babies and the change of life

Hormonal problems and infertility

At some point it will affect us all (or we may have already gone through it): the change of life. Women naturally have more problems at this time, yet men also often undergo hormonal and metabolic changes in the autumn of their lives. It is actually a natural process and an important stage in the development of every individual. Many people today tend to regard it as a degenerative process which does not chime with the dream of eternal youth propagated in the media.

Conventional medicine used to treat the change of life almost as a disease: when hormone production tails off, they are simply topped up artificially and, in this way, the person's original state can be maintained for many years.

It is understandable that some women who suffer very badly from hot flushes, outbreaks of sweating, dry mucous membranes and depressive moods have wanted to seek help in the form of this medication. Hormones were also prescribed for years, however, for patients not under any particular psychological strain - as a preventive measure to protect against heart disease and osteoporosis.

Now gynaecologists are more hesitant. For one thing, there is evidence of an increased risk of cancer after taking hormones for a prolonged period. Holistic therapists had never been fond of automatically administering hormones and an increasing number of women are now sceptical and refusing to take hormones. They are looking for alternative methods: homeopathy, phytotherapy, acupuncture and, naturally, bioresonance therapy. There are very effective bioresonance programs which have already helped a great many women (and men).

46-year-old S. W. had suffered for years from thyroid disease (Hashimoto's thyroiditis), endometriosis and high blood pressure. She came for treatment because she had currently been complaining of **hot flushes and difficulty sleeping** for five months. She was treated with bioresonance weekly for four weeks and then twice a month. After that her hot flushes and problems sleeping disappeared.

Bioresonance babies and the change of life

49-year-old G. H. came to our practice due to outbreaks of sweating, weight loss and insomnia. In addition to hormone imbalance, kinesiological testing revealed an intolerance of wheat and spelt.

An initial series of treatments dealt with the food intolerances as well as the hormone programs. The patient was symptom-free after four treatments.

Three months later she again complained about **menopausal symptoms**, this time with extreme tiredness, racing heart and dizziness. She was given the hormone programs three more times at weekly intervals, then three more times at monthly intervals. Once again the symptoms completely disappeared.

In additional to menopausal symptoms there are a range of other diseases and health problems where hormone imbalance plays a causal role. These include puberty problems, menstrual problems, endometriosis, fertility problems, mastopathy, problems with pregnancy and birth, symptoms following gynaecological surgery, Caesarean section, curettage, abortion and sterilisation. Yet hormonally induced migraine and hair loss also belong to this group. In addition to hormone programs, programs for removing scar interference, building up metabolism, eliminating toxins, allergy therapy, vegetative compensation and others are also used depending on the individual circumstances.

A 48-year-old nurse had been suffering for 13 years from diffuse **hair loss** and **menstrual problems**. She had come off the pill two months previously and been prescribed low dose gestagen by the gynaecologist. She came to our practice because, since then, her hair loss had increased and she suffered continuous abdominal pain.

After four bioresonance therapy sessions, performed one a week, for the first time in 13 years her hair stopped falling out and the abdominal pain had vanished. Even the oestrogen levels in her blood had improved (without taking oestrogen)!

Nowadays an increasing problem suffered by many young couples is **involuntary childlessness**. There are multiple causes. In women dysfunction of the ovaries, scars in the lower abdomen, hormonal problems and endometriosis play an important part. Allergic reactions to sperm have also been observed. The cause of the infertility often

Bioresonance babies and the change of life

lies with the man; most frequently, reduced sperm production or motility. Contamination with heavy metals, environmental toxins and also electromagnetic radiation are the suspected cause. Studies have already shown mobile phones in trouser pockets to be an additional risk factor.

The affected couple have to undergo a large number of examinations and treatments to be able to fulfil their wish for a child of their own. Alongside the considerable toll on their health and financial outlay of numerous fertilisation attempts (which unfortunately are not always successful), a few sessions of bioresonance therapy are an additional option which does not burden the couple excessively. Here too hormone programs, releasing therapy blocks, toxin elimination and allergy therapy are the main focus. Both partners are usually treated and vaginal discharge and sperm are used in the input cup of the bioresonance device. Bioresonance babies have now come into the world.

Non-medical practitioner M. G. has already helped several couples fulfil their wish for a child – using bioresonance therapy, combined with homeopathic remedies. "We want a baby and we've already tried all the medical options but 'they' can't help us. We even tried artificial insemination once." The woman had repeatedly suffered inflammation of the ovaries in the last ten years. She experienced severe period pains so that she kept having to take sick leave. Every possible version of the pill had been tried to stop these pains. She had not taken the pill for 3 _ years as they wanted to start a family. The husband had neurodermatitis and expressed a wish not to receive treatment. Nevertheless both were treated with bioresonance. The call came eight (!) weeks after the first appointment: "I'm pregnant!" Anna Viktoria was born in May 2004.

An older couple also came to the same therapist: "I have now remarried and my dream is to have a child with this husband. But I'm now 42 and am afraid of complications, especially for the child." The husband suffered from sleep apnoea and had to sleep with a breathing device. Three months after the first bioresonance therapy session the patient had a trouble-free pregnancy. Even the gynaecologist's attempts to cause panic were parried brilliantly. Marian came into the world in May 2003.

> Hormonal disorders such as menstrual problems and symptoms associated with the change of life generally improve with bioresonance therapy. Couples with fertility problems have often been helped to produce a bioresonance baby.

Problems in the mouth area

Dental conditions

What use has a dentist for a bioresonance device? Dentists who tend to operate along conventional medical lines but yet want to venture into alternative methods of treatment generally begin with **pre- and post-operative treatments** before and after dental surgery.

It has been universally reported that bioresonance greatly reduces impaired wound healing, inflammation, bleeding, bruises, lymphostasis, poor scar formation and other complications rarely occur. As with other types of surgery the dental patient is usually 'pre-treated' once before the operation to prepare their energetic system as best as possible. After the operation, bioresonance programs such as 'acute tissue processes', 'promoting wound healing', 'removal of scar interference', 'lymph activation', etc. are generally applied three or four times.

Our own sons had all four wisdom teeth extracted at the age of 17. They were obviously given pre- and post-operative treatment with bioresonance. They needed neither antibiotics nor painkillers, their cheeks were hardly swollen and everything was completely healed within a week. General and local anaesthetics can also be easily eliminated with bioresonance, which is particularly beneficial for sensitive patients.

Another area of use is **toxin elimination following removal and replacement of amalgam**. Reference has already been made to the problem of amalgam fillings in the chapter on 'toxic contamination'. But it's not only amalgam which can cause problems in the mouth or body. **Allergies and intolerance response to dental materials** play an increasing role in the appropriate care of patients.

A growing number of dentists are learning energetic test methods to be able to test patients' tolerance of materials ideally before the planned surgery. They can spare themselves and their patients a lot of trouble afterwards. Some dentists, who do not themselves carry out testing, work with appropriate doctors or non-medical practitioners and first send patients with the relevant samples for material testing.

Unfortunately patients often only come to the therapist when they are already suffering

Problems in the mouth area

symptoms in their mouth or some other part of the body. Frequently metals in gold alloys, crown teeth, prostheses, braces as well as synthetic and bonding materials are responsible. Symptoms range from vague toothache, inflammation and periodontitis to headaches, back ache, rashes, tinnitus and loss of neurological function.

One particularly striking case was a patient who came to us with facial paresis (paralysis of the facial muscles) which had persisted for several weeks. She had undergone a thorough neurological examination at the university hospital, yet this was inconclusive. If no cause is established, this is known as idiopathic facial paresis. She had previously been given new gold fillings by her dentist.

Kinesiological testing revealed a definite negative reaction to this material. She brought along samples from the dentist with which we conducted bioresonance allergy therapy. After two treatment sessions the palsy had all but disappeared.

We have also successfully treated offending material directly in the mouth 'in vivo' as no samples were available. In most cases this energetic desensitisation avoids the unpleasant and costly business of replacing the material.

In our experience palladium in gold alloys can be problematical. Since this is a toxic substance, it cannot really be made tolerable. After gold fillings containing palladium were fitted, a patient had severe itching eczema on both arms and on the upper body. An attempt at bioresonance therapy brought no improvement. In this case only complete removal of the offending fillings and subsequent energetic elimination resulted in the desired effect.

In conventional medical circles the rumour is still circulating that titanium is completely harmless and cannot trigger allergies. Yet we have already successfully treated a number of patients with a definite intolerance response to titanium! I now habitually ask all patients with vague symptoms if they had dental treatment prior to the onset of their symptoms. Many dentists do not realise what they can do to their patients with (untested) treatment.

There are cases where it is not the materials themselves which the patient doesn't tolerate. The presence of different metals together in the mouth can be problematical (e.g.

amalgam fillings next to gold crowns). Various metals lead to electric voltage and oral currents. If they exceed the recommended limits, this can result in health injuries. Some bioresonance devices are able to measure electric voltage and current and can give the therapist important information about treatment.

Periodontosis, periodontitis, aphthae and other inflammations in the mouth area are often caused by amalgam contamination, dental material which is not tolerated, dental foci but also by fungal infection, food allergies or organ diseases. These causes should be eliminated or treated before any surgery. A 44-year-old patient had been suffering for a long time from persistent bleeding of the gum at the 4th and 5th upper right teeth. Periodontal surgery was unsuccessful. The cause was the onset of a lung tumour.

Pain on biting and chewing is often caused by functional or anatomical **malposition of the temporomandibular joint** or a block in the hyoid bone. This may be indicated by teeth grinding or worn dental enamel on one side. Anatomical malposition is corrected by the dentist or orthodontist with a bite guard splint.

However, functional disorders are far more common. There is a special bioresonance method for correcting temporomandibular joint and hyoid bone blocks which has proved very effective. It requires a special roller electrode. The combination of positive oscillations and gentle massage releases all the neck and jaw muscles in no time. Osteopaths have reported that manual correction is much easier if the patient has received prior bioresonance treatment.

The temporomandibular joint is part of a locomotor system which connects the whole back and many joints through muscle chains. Malposition of the temporomandibular joint can not only cause scoliosis of the spine but also compensatory malposition of the hip joints. This can lead to the leg being functionally shortened. This malposition is only really rectified by prescribing compensating shoe inserts.

After bioresonance treatment of the temporomandibular joint the hips are usually level again and the legs of equal length! Suddenly not only the pain in the hips but the (associated) pain in the knees and ankles has disappeared, as if by magic. A seminar participant registered for a demonstration of bioresonance treatment of the temporomandibular joint as she ground her teeth. The next day she reported that, for the first time in

Problems in the mouth area

15 years, she had been able to go down the stairs without any pain in her knees.

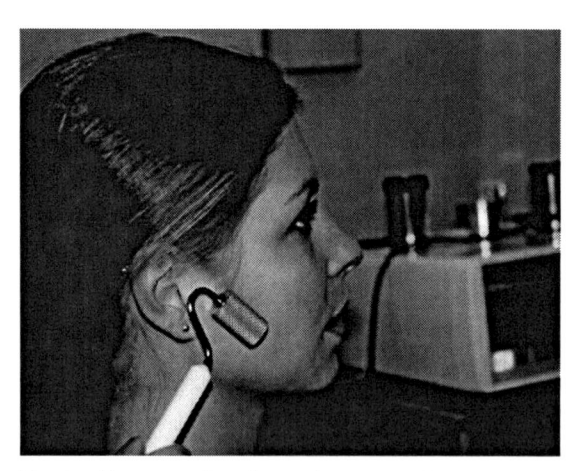

Fig. 24: Using a roller electrode to treat the temporomandibular joint.

Temporomandibular joint blocks also play a large part in migraine, tension headaches, chronic pain in the back of the neck and tinnitus. In some cases braces may be a useful way of correcting dental malposition in children. Migraine-type headaches and backache are often experienced as side-effects. A change in pressure (possibly also material intolerance) may play a part here. Bioresonance therapy was able to significantly alleviate the symptoms here too.

Holistic dentists have understood that the mouth is not isolated from the rest of the body but that it is constantly exchanging energy with the remaining organism. Dentists have known for decades that dental foci could spread bacteria and, in the pre-penicillin age, bacterially-induced valvular heart disease, nephritis and articular rheumatism were not uncommon.

We still occasionally encounter elderly patients whose teeth were all taken out to eliminate foci. In most cases it is not the material, e.g. bacterial or viral spread via the blood stream and lymph tracts which plays a crucial part but energetic remote action. In neural therapy teeth suspected of causing problems are injected with a local anaesthetic (e.g. procaine) to diagnose (or treat) the remote action on physical symptoms. This became well-known through the (unfortunately only now rarely occurring) 'flash phenomenon'. The German doctors Ferdinand and Walter Huneke demonstrated that, by injecting an interference field or dental focus, arthritic pain or other symptoms disappear immediately.

The father of electroacupuncture, Reinhold Voll, developed a complete system of energetic connections between acupuncture meridians, teeth, organs, joints and vertebral segments. Kinesiology also recognises connections between teeth and muscles which are, in turn, assigned to particular acupuncture meridians. It is astounding how often these energetic connections prove to be true in practice. And it is just as astounding when

Problems in the mouth area

symptoms improve at one point on the body although a completely different point was treated due to the energetic connections.

The energetic interrelation between tooth and organ operates in both directions. A diseased tooth can cause physical symptoms; a diseased organ can lead to dental problems. Strictly speaking, we are dealing here with the odonton, which includes the jaw area and tooth socket, tooth and root. The odonton is still present and active when the tooth has been removed.

A patient came for bioresonance treatment due to recurrent eczema in her face and upper body. Despite thoroughly tested allergy therapy she endured severe initial exacerbation each time and success was only short-lived. When searching for the focus, two dental foci in the lower left jaw kept testing as causing energetic interference. Only when the dentist had removed a cyst and chronic inflammation and the area was treated again energetically, were further bioresonance treatments effective and did the eczema disappear.

In more straightforward cases dental foci can be eliminated simply with bioresonance therapy. If more extensive clean-up or removal and replacement is required, the involvement of the dentist is requested. It often happens that a tooth tests negative energetically and the dentist cannot find anything abnormal either in the X-ray or clinical examination. If the patient insists on intervention, a chronic inflammatory focus is often discovered beneath the intact crown. Dental clean-up improves the patient's problems. Potential interference fields with possible remote action include dead teeth, root-treated teeth, cysts, granuloma and chronic inflammations.

In the case described, the dental focus acted remotely on the energy levels in organs or joints. According to dentists operating holistically, the inverse situation occurs just as frequently. The tooth is part of a complex energetic system and coupled via the meridians to organ functions, interacting continuously with them and involved in various compensatory mechanisms. As the weakest link in the regulatory system the tooth can be the first to display warning symptoms (e.g. toothache) or develop a compensatory inflammation if the system is overstretched. It is like a fuse which blows when the domestic electricity system is overloaded.

Problems in the mouth area

In our practice we have quite often found that, while treating an organ with bioresonance, a previously latent inflammatory tooth responds or even reacts violently. The latent smouldering inflammation had become an acute process and so required dental treatment. This was then an important step in the healing process, however.

The dentist S. S. reports of cases of vague pain and inflammations in the mouth area for which no cause could be determined by means of conventional medicine or dentistry. Energetic testing frequently revealed functional or organic disorders of which neither the GP nor the patient were aware.

A 25-year-old patient suffered from recurrent pain in tooth upper left 7. He also had bite problems in this area and his fillings kept losing their marginality after a short time. Energetic testing revealed an acute inflammatory process in the stomach meridian and infection of the stomach with the bacteria Helicobacter pylori (according to conventional medicine, this pathogen is often responsible for chronic gastritis and ulcers). After appropriate therapy the dental problems had also disappeared.

A 68-year-old patient suffered from burning pain with local mucosal changes in the area of tooth upper left 4, which had been previously extracted however. Not even an expert could determine the cause of the problem. The ampoule 'Degenerated cells lungs' from the tumour test set (see chapter 'Degenerated cell growth') resonated! Once the therapy was completed the mucosal changes disappeared and the patient was symptom-free. Dr S. S. points out that an organic pathological process is almost always present if a tooth or class of teeth relapses despite careful curettage or other treatment.

> Dentists use the bioresonance method to provide biophysical support for surgery and with amalgam poisoning, temporomandibular joint blocks and for dental material which the patient does not tolerate. Holistic therapists consider the energetic links between teeth and organs.

Our four-legged and feathered friends

Cases from veterinary medicine

Bioresonance for animals? If you think I'm going to tell you about horses, then you're quite right. The success that has been achieved in treating horses, dogs, cats, hamsters, birds and many other of man's four-legged and feathered companions with bioresonance is almost incredible.

Many vets, both conventional and naturopathic, have now discovered the benefits of bioresonance. Not to mention the many human therapists who not only successfully treat their patients and themselves but their pets too, if necessary. Animals generally respond much better and faster to therapy than people. They probably lack the sceptical attitude of some human patients who sometimes refuse therapy. They intuitively sense what is good for them. When the right therapy is running, they stand or lie on the ground or examination couch quite calmly and relaxed with the electrodes in position. Once the therapy is over or is no longer appropriate, they become unsettled or stand up to leave the place where therapy is being performed.

As for the argument that bioresonance is purely placebo therapy, they would probably laugh if they could. Often just a few therapy sessions are sufficient to bring about successful treatment. We also observe similarly rapid reactions in infants and small children to those witnessed in animals.

Positive treatment of animals has been reported for allergies, infectious diseases, paralysis and many other disorders specific to animals. We also encounter similar conditions to those found in human medicine: therapy blocks, interference fields, chronic infection with toxins and germs.

Just like people, animals are forced to deal with allergies to food or environmental factors with increasing frequency. Some animal species are particularly sensitive to radiation. Dogs quickly become sick if their baskets are placed on a watercourse intersection and it is almost impossible to treat horses if their stall is affected by geopathic stress. In the past, farmers called the water diviner if a cow in their barn did not give milk. As well as

Our four-legged and feathered friends

those who avoid radiation, there are also animals which feel particularly good in interference zones. These include cats, as well as ants!

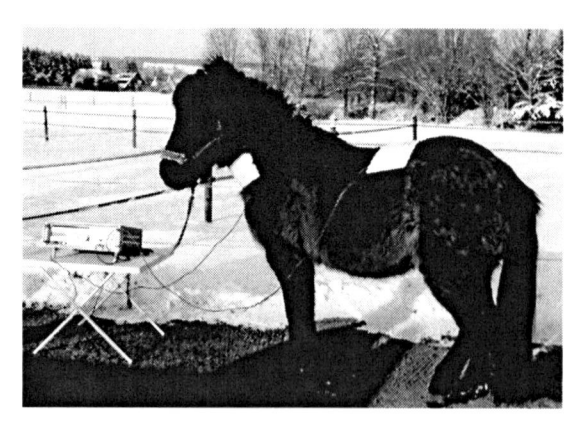

Fig. 25: The Icelandic mare Kira was cured of her laminitis with bioresonance.

Energetic testing is usually performed on animals by means of the tensor technique, either directly or on a drop of blood. It is also possible to test using kinesiology via a surrogate person positioned between the animal and the device. Electrode positioning is straightforward. The input electrode is generally placed on the back, the back of the neck or on the part of the body requiring treatment. The modulation mat serving as output is placed on the lower back area of larger animals, while smaller animals simply lie on top of it. 'Informed' fluids are added to the animal's food and the 'informed metal chip' can be hung around its neck.

Horses are often very valuable animals not only from a material perspective; there is a strong emotional bond with the owner. Some animal lovers spend a lot of money on the wellbeing and health of their animals. Therapy is usually carried out in the stable. The flexible input electrode is usually placed on the back of the neck with extra long cables while the modulation mat, serving as output, lies on the lower back near the kidneys.

It is very impressive when a huge animal stands quite calmly in the stable and begins to sway slightly or yawn at the tiny therapeutic impulses. Afterwards it should be allowed to rest for a while.

A 17-year-old Trakehner mare had always been a poor eater. Although she was given twice the amount of food of other horses, she did not eat much and looked thin and run down. The animal also reacted to any type of stress by refusing food. When the therapist R. L. entered the stable to treat the horse, it was still standing in the stall after an afternoon ride wet and trembling with its head hanging. Its full feeding trough had not been touched.

Testing revealed a **straw allergy.** During the first treatment program the animal stopped sweating and trembling. After the third therapy program the horse was led into the stall where, to the owner's astonishment, it immediately began to eat until the trough was empty. The owner was advised to switch from straw to sawdust to cover the floor of the stall. A second therapy session followed two weeks later. The animal was now already totally different, almost always ate all the food in its trough, had gained weight and seemed more stable.

Six months later the animal's general state of health was still very good, it was eating sufficient food and its weight was normal. It could be fed straw once again, without provoking a reaction.

A colt was born with no human intervention. The vet who was called out shortly afterwards diagnosed **paralysis of the back legs** and tail root, probably caused by the fall at birth. That day the animal had to be bottle-fed as it could not stand to drink. The vet noticed from the X-ray that the first two cervical vertebrae were dislocated and advised having the foal put to sleep.

The animal was two days old when R.. E. began bioresonance therapy. After the first therapy session the foal could already lift its little tail. The following day it could already stand unsupported, yet had to be lifted up for the next two days. After the second treatment session it took its first independent steps. It was, however, still unable to lift or turn its head. After the third bioresonance therapy session the foal moved normally, just slightly slower than its contemporaries. It was also now able to drink from its mother unaided. After three months the animal's behavioural development was completely normal for its age and it moved quite normally in all three types of gait.

The twelve-year-old dappled stallion 'Nevado' had two tumours, larger than fists, in the abdominal area. One tumour was near the navel, the second larger tumour was at the point where the girth would normally be fastened so that the horse could no longer be ridden. Conventional medical diagnosis: **equine sarcoid**, a malignant soft tissue tumour caused by papillomavirus. Three vets had already treated the animal, to no avail. Surgery was not an option.

When the animal therapist S. B. saw the extremely emaciated horse for the first time, she threw her hands up in horror: "I wouldn't have given five pounds for the horse" and she

Our four-legged and feathered friends

told the owner she didn't hold out any hope that bioresonance would be able to achieve anything. The owner was very enthusiastic about the bioresonance method, however, as she had had extremely positive personal experience of it and wanted to try everything to improve the animal's lot.

Treating the animal was not initially easy as it must have been in considerable pain. The horse wouldn't allow anyone to touch it and moved away when anyone came near. Tensor testing revealed multiple infections with fungi, bacteria, parasites and viruses. With considerable patience on the part of the owner and therapist, Nevado allowed the therapies to be applied. Its kidneys, liver and intestines were stabilised, yeast and mould fungi and also liver fluke were eliminated. Next the Borrelia and Staphylococcus infections were treated and finally the papillomavirus in combination with herpes virus. After four months Nevado was already much better. He had put on weight and the tumours were visibly smaller.

After a total of 30 bioresonance therapy sessions the tumours had healed completely and the enthusiastic owner could ride Nevado once more.

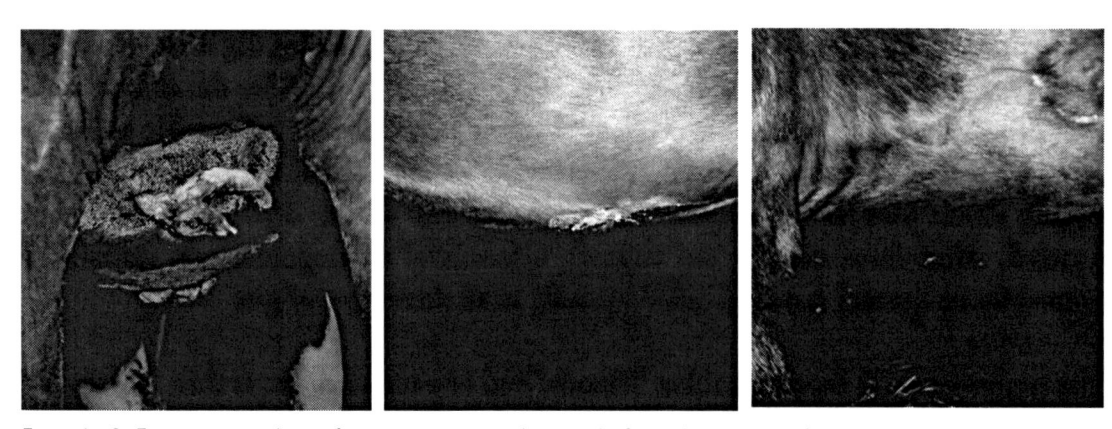

Fig. 26-28: Equine sarcoid, a soft tissue tumour in horses, before, during and after bioresonance therapy.

It is not only amateur animal owners who are fans of the bioresonance method. It has now also found favour in livestock management circles. Farmers and breeders are increasingly disinclined to feed their animals chemical drugs and are placing growing importance on 'gentle' treatment methods. A farmer's best **breeding boar** (three years old) lay in its stall and no longer stirred. It had an abnormal swelling on its back, known as **banana disease**, an inflammation of the large extensor muscle on the back. Consequently it was no longer able to mate. The concern here was to bring about genuine healing and not simply reduce the swelling using drugs with the risk of subsequent total necrosis of the muscle. The farmer announced he was prepared to try bioresonance therapy. The evening after the first treatment the swelling had actually subsided to such an extent that the boar was able to walk again. After two days it was fully fit once more. It had absolutely no symptoms when mating which is not always the case when traditional methods are used.

Small animals, especially dogs and cats, are often a definite part of the family. Children, parents and grandparents feel sympathy when the pet is unwell and will try everything to prevent a family drama. There are now numerous fans of the bioresonance method amongst this group.

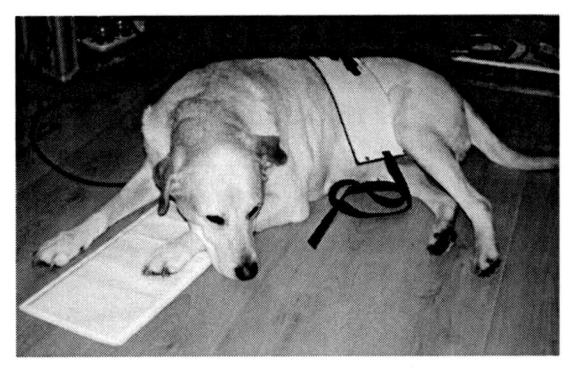

Fig. 29: Labrador bitch Mira is treated for back pain.

Dogs generally lie calmly on the bioresonance device's modulation mat until the therapy session is over. The vet Dr. med. vet. M. V. treated an eleven-year-old Irish Setter which had suffered severe itching, hair loss and digestive problems for years. The animal had already been treated with antibiotics, homeopathy and its own blood without success.

The resonance test revealed **food allergies** to beef and maize. Beef was removed from its diet and the dog was treated with bioresonance four times. At the same time medication to regulate the intestines was also administered. The itching vanished and the animal's digestion returned to normal. It could tolerate beef once more and the maize allergy also disappeared without being specifically treated. The dog was still completely symptom-free eight months later and had grown a full glossy coat of fur.

A ten-year-old Yorkshire Terrier bitch suffered **spastic paralysis** and was brought to the practice of Mag. vet A.. J. The dog was completely stiff and could no longer stand up at all. After three bioresonance treatments at intervals of two to three days the dog was rushing around as before without the slightest physical disability.

A female crossbreed gun dog was already on heat for the first time at the age of six months. At eight months she was showing all the symptoms of a **false pregnancy** including swollen mammary glands. The vet A. J. treated the animal three times with bioresonance. After that she got over everything and the milk stopped without any hormones, to which dogs are often highly sensitive, being administered. The animal was in excellent condition.

Leishmaniasis is a parasitic infectious tropical disease in dogs which, according to conventional medicine, is incurable. It is a serious disorder in which the dog may lose all its fur. If diagnosed with this condition, the animal must take medication throughout its entire life. Leishmaniasis is not considered to be curable, merely treatable.

The vet S. M. had already successfully treated several dogs with this disease. The Labrador crossbreed bitch Gipsy was a holiday souvenir from a trip to Greece. When giving the necessary vaccination, the Greek vet noticed bald patches in the animal's fur and the blood test confirmed the suspected diagnosis of leishmaniasis. The dog was treated five times with bioresonance without the usual drug treatment. Its fur began to grow back within three weeks. A further lab test was subsequently conducted. The result was absolutely incredible, but true: Gipsy was leishmaniasis-negative! The whole family was beside itself with joy.

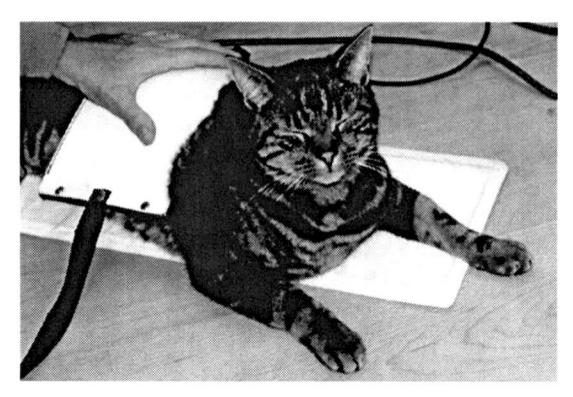

Fig. 30: Moghli enjoys the bioresonance therapy.

Cats also respond very well to bioresonance treatment. The vet Dr med. vet. J. R. treated a female house cat with **infectious cat flu**. Its eyes had been stuck together and nose blocked for a long time. The animal frequently sneezed, appeared tired and its fur was dull. In the meantime the animal had been treated with 'Jungtiersuspension' [injectable medication for young animals] but this had proved unsuccessful. After two bioresonance therapy sessions at intervals of two days an improvement was already noticeable. The nose and eyes were no longer as blocked, although the animal still needed to sneeze frequently. Three days later the owner called to report that the cat was well again and romping around happily.

Miou, a sterilised female house cat, had already been suffering for over six weeks from a **urinary tract infection** causing considerable pain on urinating. She tried to pass water six or seven times a day and had to squeeze hard in doing so, yet only produced a few drops. The owner had already visited two veterinary practices, had the urine tested and antibiotics prescribed. Yet the symptoms only disappeared for a brief spell.

Dr med. vet. Sch.'s testing revealed mercury as the main problem, probably from thiomersal, an inactive ingredient in vaccines, as well as parasitic infection with Schistosoma. After the first bioresonance session where the contaminating factors were eliminated and kidneys offered energetic support, the cat lying on the modulation mat had already relaxed visibly. The second therapy session took place after six days. Three days later the owner called to report that the cat was much better and was no longer displaying any symptoms. After the third session Miou was restored to full health and lively. No further recurrence had occurred even three years after the therapy.

A two-year-old **guinea pig** had been suffering for a month from severe hair loss and had lost a great deal of weight. The usual treatment with antifungal medication had proved unsuccessful and the owner had almost given up hope of a cure. Dr med. vet. M. K. diagnosed an **allergy to hay**. The animal was treated with three bioresonance therapy sessions at two day intervals. Four months later the guinea pig was still not displaying any symptoms. Its coat was glossy and the animal had a good appetite.

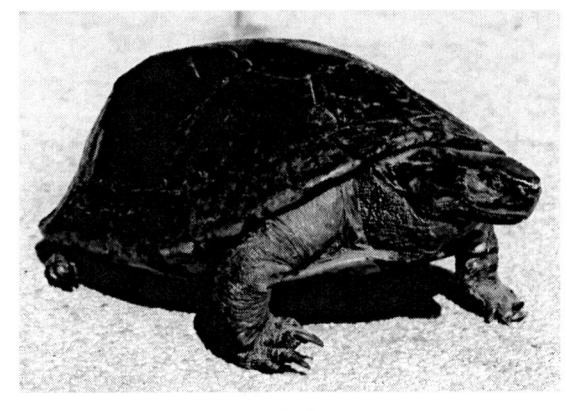

Fig. 31: Even reptiles benefit from bioresonance therapy.

The small one-year-old **terrapin** had woken up normally from hibernation yet had stopped eating after a month and was completely listless. With an open mouth it was gasping for air: diagnosis - **inflammation of the lungs**. Antibiotic treatment proved unsuccessful. Dr med. vet. M. V. treated the animal with bioresonance three times at three day intervals. After this the terrapin ate normally once again and no longer displayed any symptoms.

Our four-legged and feathered friends

The bioresonance therapist E. B. has lived in Dubai for over 20 years. One day one of her acquaintances, a sheikh, asked her whether the bioresonance method could also be used on falcons. Two of his Saker **falcons** had had problems with **bumblefoot** (ulcers on the ball of the foot) for a long time. The birds were extremely valuable but could no longer be used for hunting. The ulcers on their feet were so large that they even had difficulty standing. They were eating very little and were so weak that they were no longer able to fly.

The owner, who bred falcons, had already lost several birds to bumblefoot. Conventional medicine could do nothing. The sheikh was at first extremely sceptical and initially brought just one falcon for treatment.

Just a few days after the first bioresonance therapy session the bird's condition had already improved and the wound was beginning to close. The owner quickly brought a second bird suffering with the disease, which also had an inflamed eye and allergic respiratory problems. The treatments were very quick and easy and progressed without any problems. The breeder was impressed and astonished that everything went so smoothly, causing the birds no stress and that the symptoms had already disappeared after just three weeks. He immediately recommended the method to other falcon breeders.

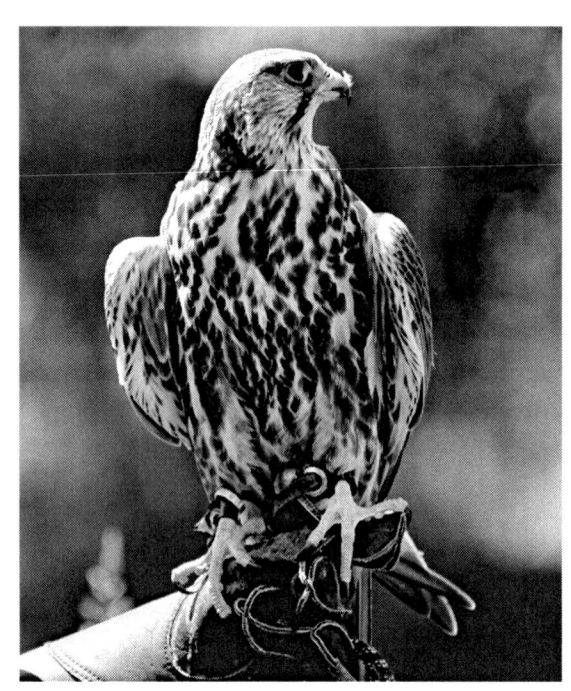

Fig. 32: Valuable hunting falcons were cured of bumblefoot.

There is one creature which is not receptive to the bioresonance method: **the inner demon**. And that is something you have to tackle if you want to learn and use a new treament method. Fortunately there is no shortage of help available for newcomers who can fall back on a wealth of experience gathered by long-standing therapists.

Our four-legged and feathered friends

> Both large and small animals respond very quickly to the bioresonance method. Even conditions which are considered incurable, such as leishmaniasis in dogs, respond to treatment.

What evidence is available?

Efficacy and evidence-based studies

"The efficacy of bioresonance is not scientifically proven." This often quoted argument may have been valid back in the early 1990s. However, the situation has now changed fundamentally. A large number of scientific studies have been published in the last few years which provide conclusive proof of the efficacy of this method and give confirmed critics pause for thought. Even the Munich higher regional court had to bow to the scientific evidence in a recent ruling, following a five-year legal dispute. As a result it is now lawfully permissible to advertise that the bioresonance method "is able to diagnose and treat allergies". It has been a long hard road getting to this point, however.

Many scientists insist on **double blind trials** as the only valid proof of efficacy of a therapeutic method. These have now become the standard requirement for introducing new medicines. Double blind trials have become the 'golden calf' of objective natural science and some scientists believe that this is the only way to obtain a usable result. It is often forgotten in this, however, that there are certainly many other study profiles which are scientifically recognised. Double blind trials are seldom conducted in the strongholds of research, the universities. Most doctoral and post-doctoral theses tend to be cohort or case control studies, longitudinal studies, studies involving animal experimentation and mechanistic model studies. Without these fundamental baseline studies, new drugs and methods of therapy would probably never be developed.

Why are these double blind trials so highly regarded and why are none yet available for bioresonance? If a therapist reports that their treatment has produced a positive result in one or more patients, critics tend to consider this pure chance, the placebo effect, a spontaneous recovery or an incorrect diagnosis. This criticism is quite understandable if it is a matter of one individual case. If I have successfully treated a patient with a particular method (medication or some other means), I never know whether the improvement was the result of my therapeutic intervention or whether the patient would have got better without any treatment.

Patients often do recover spontaneously from their medical conditions, in other words

What evidence is available?

without the therapist's intervention and it was pure chance that the therapy and improvement coincided. If, however, I repeatedly observe improvements in a large number of patients after a series of treatments and with disorders where spontaneous recovery seldom occurs, even the most persistent critics are at a loss to explain the statistics. It is then sometimes claimed that the initial diagnosis (generally made by the therapist themselves) must have been incorrect as otherwise there could no explanation for this improvement.

And then there is the famous **placebo effect** (from the Latin placebo = I please). "Faith can move mountains" and the mind controls (many) bodily functions. There are even a number of scientific studies of this placebo effect.

Patients who firmly believe in their own recovery, in the therapist and in the medicine or the treatment are cured far more frequently, statistically speaking, than those whose attitude tends to be more critical. What is more: if the doctor or non-medical practitioner also firmly believes in their treatment and conveys this to the patient, either consciously or subconsciously, it works even better. Rituals play a large part in this. For the primitive people's medicine men it was drums and prayers; for today's medicine men it's tablets, injections, infusions or therapy devices.

In the case of chronic disorders, in particular, between 30 and 50% of patients recover or see their symptoms improve at least, simply by taking sugar pills and saline solution with no pharmaceutical efficacy, in other words as a result of faith and ritual.

If less than 50% of patients recover as a result of administering a particular medication, it is disputed whether this medication really does produce an effect independently. And this is precisely the reason why double blind trials were developed. The aim is to try to rule out placebo effects, chance and spontaneous recovery as far as possible to enable the efficacy of a substance or a method to be assessed as objectively as possible. This is particularly difficult in the field of medicine since relatively large numbers of patients with the same circumstances rarely occur. Even patients suffering from the same medical condition often differ widely in other parameters such as age, gender, constitution, secondary diagnoses, additional medication, etc.

And now here's the formula for a double blind trial.

What evidence is available?

Take as many patients as possible (one hundred to several thousand) with a conclusive diagnosis determined by conventional medical methods. Let's assume we are dealing with patients with high blood pressure (hypertension) and a new blood pressure medication (antihypertensive agent) is being tested.

The patients are divided into two groups. One half are given the right medication (verum), the other half a sugar pill which looks exactly the same (placebo). Patients are assigned to groups at random (randomised).

If only the patient does not know what he is getting, this is a **single blind trial**. If the doctor does not know what he is giving either, then it is a **double blind trial**.

At the end of a predetermined period, the reduction in blood pressure in the two groups is compared. The blood pressure of many patients in the placebo group will naturally also have fallen and many in this group will even complain of side-effects! Only if the blood pressure of considerably more patients (a statistically significant number) in the verum group effectively falls is the efficacy of this new medication proven. The larger the number of patients in both groups, the more conclusive the result statistically.

Many scientists are now demanding this type of proof of efficacy through double blind trials not just for conventional medicines but also for naturopathic remedies and for alternative therapies. And here the problem for naturopathy becomes evident. While conventional medication is administered **based on the diagnosis** (all the study group members with hypertension are given the same antihypertensive agent), the therapies of most naturopathic methods are generally **individual**.

In classic homeopathy every person with high blood pressure will be given a different remedy based on their constitution and other circumstances of their symptoms. In acupuncture the points to needle are also selected according to constitution and accompanying symptoms.

In bioresonance, when patients are affected by multiple factors, the programs required are often tested out using an energetic method of diagnosis. Therapy is always individual and no therapist with their own practice is keen to conduct placebo therapy. A single blind trial would be conceivable under certain conditions. A double blind trial, where even

What evidence is available?

the therapist does not know whether they are administering the effective treatment, is virtually impossible.

But there has now also been some movement in the naturopathy camp. Proof of efficacy from double blind trials is now available for **complex homeopathic remedies**, which can also be used on the basis of a diagnosis. Several meta-analyses[18] from the last 20 years have been published in which various homeopathy studies were compared and assessed. Some of these studies proved that **homeopathic medications** were more effective than placebos while others could not find evidence of any difference. Authors always accuse those in the opposing camp of irregularities in the selection of studies. A generally accepted scientific solution does not yet appear to be in sight.

Between 2001 and 2005 a multi-centre effectiveness study of over fifty thousand patients was conducted for **acupuncture** at the request and with the financial support of the health insurance funds. Statistically significant improvements, equivalent to those obtained with drug treatment, were seen for the indications "pain in the lumbar spine" and "arthritis of the knee". As a result, these indications were included amongst those eligible for reimbursement by the health insurance providers. Some practices also conducted a single blind trial with placebo acupuncture in which they needled patients at points other than the traditional acupuncture points. No statistically significant difference was observed here compared with the patient group which was correctly needled. It was debated whether many points other than the traditional meridians could also be effective.

And now to **bioresonance**. Scientific studies are usually carried out in laboratories, research institutions, practices or in universities. In Germany the universities represent the highest scientific authority. Appropriate committees made up of professors and researchers specify what the "current state of scientific knowledge" is at that particular point in time.

Expert assessments conducted in universities usually form the basis for the higher courts'

---

[18] Shan A. et al.: Are the clinical effects of homeopathy placebo effects? Comparative study of placebo-controlled trials of homeopathy and allopathy, 366: 726-32, Lancet 2005; in addition: Linde et al., Meta-analysis with 89 studies, Lancet 1997; Kleijnen et al., Meta-analysis with 107 studies, British Medical Journal, 1991; Linde and Melchart, Meta-analysis with 32 studies, Journal of Alternative and Complementary Medicine, 1998.

What evidence is available?

rulings in legal disputes. As a result they bear a heavy responsibility towards the general public.

You would think that universities would be driven by a keen passion for research and that new, possibly pioneering ideas would be investigated with academic curiosity using objective criteria and then confirmed or rejected.

All the more astonishing then that many therapeutic approaches from the world of naturopathy seem to be completely ignored. Absolutely no notice is taken of positive experience gained from actual practice especially if the ideas on which it is based do not fit in with the prevailing (but, in fact, outdated) world view. And university courses on these topics? Currently out of the question!

Research is **expensive**. Pharmaceutical firms invest millions in research and in studies proving the efficacy of new medicines. Small and medium-sized businesses don't have the funds for this. In recent years the law has required fresh licenses to be obtained for many drugs whereby their efficacy had to be investigated and proven in new trials. As a result many tried and tested natural remedies were removed from the market since most small firms did not have the necessary financial resources.

And who is conducting research into bioresonance now?

First of all, enthusiastic therapists who observe successful treatment in their practices and, fired with idealism, laboriously record cases. Individual case reports do not by any means constitute scientific proof. However, it is not so easy to ignore hundreds and thousands of individual case reports.

In 2005 a manufacturer of bioresonance devices conducted a survey in which 538 doctors and non-medical practitioners who use this method in their practices took part. Treatment of 684,366(!) patients was evaluated in the process. 50.5% of these indicated they were symptom-free, 31.0% reported a definite and 11.7% a slight improvement. Only 5.8% of cases reported no improvement and 1.0% a deterioration.

Bioresonance led to freedom from symptoms in 46% of 241,664 cases which had been treated exhaustively with conventional medicine. A definite improvement was observed

What evidence is available?

in 34.0% and a slight improvement in 13.1% of cases. Only 6.2% of patients could not be helped.

Dr Rummel established a society in which all the therapists treat their patients according to his standardised allergy therapy. This has now provided over 20,000 positive case records. No conventional medical practitioner can ignore figures such as these!

Some doctors conducted **effectiveness studies**, interviewed the patients treated and analysed the results statistically. Hospitals have stated that they are not yet ready for this type of research, at least not in Europe. **But they are in China!**

It almost sounds like a parody of the history of medicine. A method is discovered in Germany based, in part, on the teachings of Chinese medicine, dating back thousands of years. While this method is largely ignored in Germany, it is exported back to China. There it is not only applied with enthusiasm but scientific studies are also conducted in hospitals. These then help this method gain recognition in Germany. A positive effect of globalisation.

In December 2004 my wife and I held a seminar in connection with a bioresonance congress in the city of Xian, famous for the excavations of the terracotta army. This was attended by over a hundred doctors and professors from throughout China. We had originally assumed that clinics practising Traditional Chinese Medicine would be interested in this method. But this was not the case. Several hundred Bicom devices can be found exclusively in modern hospitals where otherwise Western medicine is practised. Private doctor's practices do not yet exist in China, as they do here. The Chinese are curious and pragmatic. For a start, any device manufactured in Germany is interesting. And then they give it a try.

If it works, then they carry on using it. If it doesn't, it's a flop. And they didn't just carry on using bioresonance; they even conducted several **scientific studies.**

There are some advantages in this regard in China, compared with Europe. Salaries are still low, there appear to be sufficient funds available and there are also sufficient patients. We visited a large hospital in Xian. Bioresonance had its own department and a member of staff treated patients with the bioresonance method from morning till night. All the

What evidence is available?

applications and results were meticulously recorded. These are obviously ideal conditions for studies on relatively large patient groups. The astonishing results are described later on.

In Europe scientific research on bioresonance has been conducted, amongst other places, in laboratories. Here experiments took place on nutrient solutions, cell cultures, blood samples, flies and tadpoles. The aim was to demonstrate that the bioresonance device does, in fact, produce oscillations which have an effect on biological systems outside the human body. They are described as **in vitro** or **animal experimentation**.

The purpose of a scientific study is to demonstrate the truth. So the findings of all the studies on the same topic should tend to display the same results. The reality is quite different however. There are studies published which have supposedly proved a fact and, two years later, you can read studies which claim exactly the opposite. Who is right then? You only have to think of the ideal cholesterol level; the recommendations change every year. Were these studies all of the same standard or were there good studies and not so good? Who discovered the truth, or to put it better, how high is the probability (or evidence) that the research got as close as possible to the truth?

Some years ago the **American Heart Association** looked for a solution to this dilemma. They introduced a classification system for scientific studies based on **levels of evidence**. This is an 8 level system (see table) intended to evaluate the quality of a study's evidence. Accordingly, evidence level 1 would be a study which has the highest likelihood of reflecting the claimed truth. This equates to a study of the highest scientific standard and is virtually regarded as proof. This includes the **statistically significant, randomised, controlled double blind trials** or **meta-analyses** described earlier. With level 8 the probability that the result is right is still heavily disputed. This group includes rational assumptions. All other forms of study lie between levels 2 and 7.

For some years doctors in medical practices and hospitals have been urged to practise evidence-based medicine. This means that, where possible, only methods and medications should be used for which level 1 and 2 studies exist. However this severely limits doctors' freedom to select therapy and work based on their therapeutic experience.

What evidence is available?

Level 1	Statistically significant randomised controlled trials or meta-analyses with statistically significant results	Meta-analyses of multiple randomised controlled trials with homogeneous and statistically significant effects from therapy or with heterogeneous results which are, on the whole, still nevertheless statistically significant
Level 2	Not statistically significant randomised controlled trials or meta-analyses, not statistically significant meta-analyses of inconsistent randomised controlled trials	Meta-analyses of multiple randomised controlled trials with consistent effects from therapy in individual trials, which are not statistically significant however; meta-analyses of multiple randomised controlled trials with heterogeneous effects from therapy which are not statistically significant
Level 3	Prospective, controlled but non-randomised cohort studies	Prospective trials on a cohort of patients who are not randomised as regards intervention; investigators usually try to establish a control group treated at the same time or a comparison group
Level 4	Historical, non-randomised cohort or case control study	Historical non-randomised cohort studies; retrospective studies or observational studies; the investigators try to provide a control or comparison group
Level 5	Longitudinal studies of patients	Studies in which patients are included either prospectively or retrospectively in consecutive order and the effects of an intervention are observed; no control group
Level 6	Studies involving animal experimentation or mechanistic models	Animal experiments or mechanistic models

What evidence is available?

Level 7	Reasonable extrapolation of existing data; quasi-experimental design	Reasonable extrapolation with a quasi-experimental design or of existing data, collected for other purposes
Level 8	Rational assumption (general belief), historical acceptance as standard practice	Practice accords with the general feeling or has apparent validity. Handed down as standard practice prior to the requirement for scientifically validated recommendations (EBM); no new scientific findings to support a change; no indication of a negative effect

Table according to American Heart Association (AHA), modified in accordance with W.F. Dick: Evidence based emergency medicine, Anaesthetist 47, 957, 1998 and Circulation 102: 1-4, 2000.

Several **bioresonance studies** have now been assessed as level 1 and 2. A manufacturer of bioresonance devices commissioned a renowned independent institute for data analysis and study planning[19] to assess the quality of fifteen bioresonance trials and assign levels of evidence to them.

Four trials were assigned level 1, one trial level 1-2, one trial level 2, one trial level 3, four trials level 4-5 and four trials level 5. The assessor summarised these investigations as follows: "All previous trials and research studies indicate that the BICOM method not only displays statistically significant effects (in the sense of an effect demonstrable by random statistics). In a clinical context these can be interpreted as efficacy. No adverse side-effects, particularly those of a serious nature, were found in any of the trials. In principle, the studies discussed and evaluated here meet the quality standard of university research."[20]

Let's look at the most important trials designed to prove the efficacy of bioresonance in a little more detail. We make a distinction between **pre-clinical trials**, conducted on mineral solutions, cell cultures, blood components and animals and **clinical trials** on patient groups.

---

[19] Institute of Data Analysis & Study Planning, Gauting.

[20] Institute of Data Analysis & Study Planning, Gauting. Expert opinion of 9.12.2005 and 20.1.2006.

What evidence is available?

First an interesting pre-clinical trial: Can non-living systems e.g. **mineral salt** solutions react to bioresonance? An interesting experiment was conducted in Slovenia in 1998.[21] Information from an acetic acid solution was applied to a neutral mineral salt solution by means of the BRT device. The treated mineral salt solutions displayed distinct physical differences compared with the untreated specimens. The informed mineral solutions became acid, resembling the acetic acid. The pH of the informed specimens dropped slightly but significantly.

Kirlian photography (high frequency high voltage photography developed by Semyon and Valentina Kirlian) of the treated solutions revealed more intensive and stronger radiation patterns and, after drying, larger and more extensive crystals formed than in the control group.

This shows that non-material information is transmitted via the Bicom device even non-living substances can undergo physical changes. Or are even mineral salt solutions taken in by supposed placebo treatment?

Cell cultures of cancer cells were treated with bioresonance for several days. These were degenerated monocytes (a subgroup of white blood corpuscles) from a human lymphoma (lymph node cancer). After three days the malignancy parameters tended to improve. DNA synthesis and the DNA content of the cells increased by over 20%, for example.[22]

Do sick patients' blood samples change if treated with information from the blood samples of healthy patients? An interesting experiment was conducted with **human serum albumin (HSA)**, the most important protein component of blood plasma.[23] The HSA of ten healthy women was mixed and information from the mixture transferred

---

[21] Thesis at the Electrical Engineering Faculty of the University of Ljubljana; N. Rojko Vuga in Prof. A. Jeglic's research group: Untersuchung der Transduktion von Essigsäure-Information über einen elektronischen Verstärker [Investigaton into the transduction of information from acetic acid via an electronic amplifier], 1997.

[22] G. Lednyiczky: Über den Einfluss der Bioresonanztherapie auf die Kanzerogenese [On the influence of bioresonance therapy on carcinogenesis] in Niederenergetische Bioinformation [Low energy bioinformation], Viennese International Academy of Holistic Medicine, vol. 17, p. 134-137, Facultas Verlag, 1997, eds. P.C. Endler and A. Stacher.

[23] O.V. Zhalko-Titarenko et al.: Der Einfluss der BICOM Resonanz auf die strukturelle Dynamik des Serum-Albumins von Patienten mit Brustkrebs [The influence of BICOM resonance on the structural dynamics of the serum albumin of patients with breast cancer], Research Centre LEKON of the Ukrainian Academy of Science, Kiev, 1995.

What evidence is available?

with the BRT device to HSA preparations from the blood of 8 breast cancer patients. Astonishingly the treated pathological HSA protein components of the breast cancer patients began to normalise. It could be concluded from this that bioresonance has a regulating effect on the immune system.

Various parameters of the Bicom device were tested on 50,000(!) blood samples. Ten ampoules of blood from the same donor were placed in the input cup and ten ampoules of blood in the output. The **phagocytosis activity** of the white blood cells (polymorphonuclear leucocytes) was examined. Phagocytosis is the incorporation and elimination of foreign material or germs by these white blood cells.

Comprehensive testing was carried out with a broad range of different therapy settings. As the following bar chart indicates, the phagocytosis activity of the untreated control group was on average 21.1, for example. Following treatment with a bioresonance therapy program it rose to 54.7 with a single amplification of the therapy signals and to 41.7 when these were amplified 12 fold. The changes were less pronounced when the information was inverted.[24]

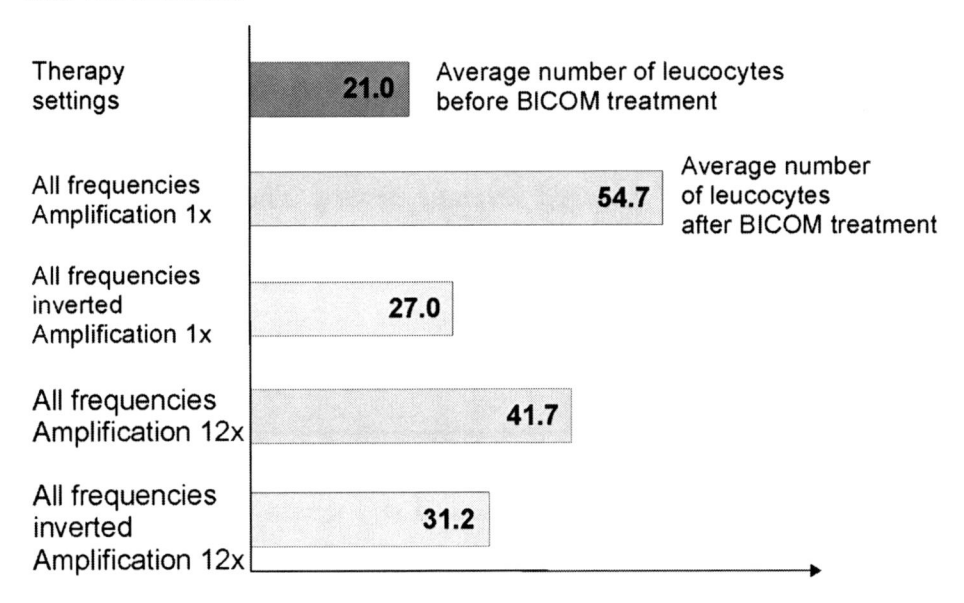

Therapy settings	Value	
(control)	21.0	Average number of leucocytes before BICOM treatment
All frequencies Amplification 1x	54.7	Average number of leucocytes after BICOM treatment
All frequencies inverted Amplification 1x	27.0	
All frequencies Amplification 12x	41.7	
All frequencies inverted Amplification 12x	31.2	

Fig. 33: Significant increase in the number of leucocytes and lymph nodes following bioresonance

---

[24] O. Osadchaya et al.: Zusammenfassende Darstellung der In-vitro-Modulation der Phagozytose-Aktivität von menschlichen polymorphkernigen Leukozyten durch BICOM Resonanz-Therapie [Summary report of in-vitro modulation of phagocytosis activity of human polymorphonuclear leucocytes by BICOM resonance therapy] in: Wissenschaftliche Studien [Scientific studies], Regumed Institut für Regulative Medizin, page 38-46, 1999.

What evidence is available?

The improvement in the quality of donor blood following bioresonance treatment in an in-vitro test is evident from the following chart, in the form of an increase in the number of active leucocytes:

Can bioresonance increase the appetite of the white blood cells and thereby improve the immune defence system?

Some animal experimentation has also been conducted in connection with bioresonance. Even heat-damaged **Drosophila larvae** (fruit fly) benefit from bioresonance therapy. **Vitality** improved significantly compared with the untreated group. Response to light stimuli and mobility normalised, survival time without food was extended.[25]

Tadpoles' transition into frogs (**metamorphosis**) is delayed if the thyroid hormone thyroxin is added to the aquarium water. This effect was also achieved when the information from the thyroxin was simply applied via the bioresonance device. Further proof that biophysical information transfer is possible and produces physiological effects. This trial was conducted **double blind** by two totally unconnected institutions in Austria and Italy.[26]

Mice contaminated with radioactivity (Chernobyl type) were also treated with bioresonance. Thymus and lymph node weight normalised in the treated group, indicating an improvement in the damaged immune system. The spleen was also observed to be enlarged which could indicate increased activity when breaking down damaged cells and blood components.[27]

The preclinical trials were all assigned the highest evidence level, **level 1**.

---

[25] G. Ledniczky: Rekonstitution der Vitalität hitzegeschädigter Drosophila-Larven mittels endogener elektromagnetischer Felder [Reconstituting the vitality of heat-damaged Drosophila larvae using endogenous electromagnetic fields], in: Niederenergetische Bioinformation [Low energy bioinformation], series vol. 17, p. 122-134, Facultas Verlag Vienna, 1997, eds. P. C. Endler and A. Stacher.

[26] P. C. Endler et al.: Übertragung von Molekül-Information mittels Bioresonanz-Gerät (BICOM) im Amphibienversuch [Transfer of molecular information via bioresonance device (BICOM) in tests on amphibians], Erfahrungsheilkunde, Heidelberg, 3, p. 186-192, 1995.

[27] D. Sakkarov et al.: Untersuchung zur Rekonstitution des Immunsystems radioaktiv kontaminierter Mäuse mittels BICOM Resonanz-Therapie [Investigation of the reconstitution of the immune system of mice contaminated with radioactivity by means of BICOM bioresonance therapy] Wissenschaftliche Studien [Scientific studies], Regumed Institut für Regulative Medizin, 1999, page 48 -55.

What evidence is available?

Thymus: increase in lymphocytes

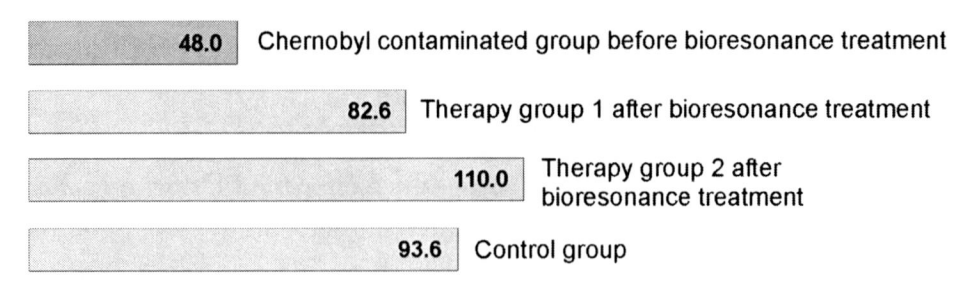

- 48.0 — Chernobyl contaminated group before bioresonance treatment
- 82.6 — Therapy group 1 after bioresonance treatment
- 110.0 — Therapy group 2 after bioresonance treatment
- 93.6 — Control group

Spleen: increase in lymphocytes

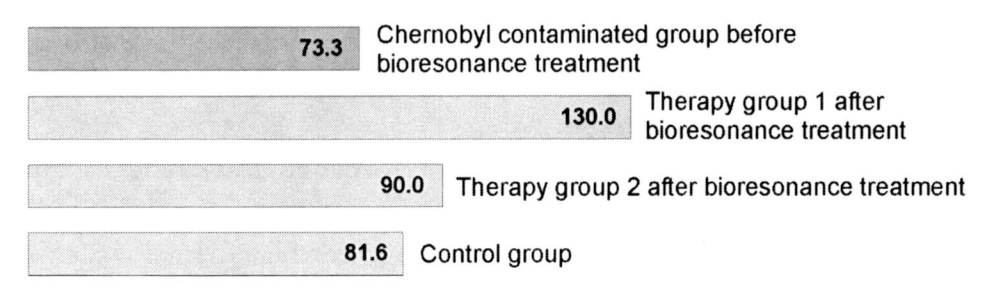

- 73.3 — Chernobyl contaminated group before bioresonance treatment
- 130.0 — Therapy group 1 after bioresonance treatment
- 90.0 — Therapy group 2 after bioresonance treatment
- 81.6 — Control group

Therapy settings:

Group 1: frequency sweep 18 s, inverted, amplification 0.8 and frequency 870 Hz, amplification H = 0.1 and Di = 0.5 fold

Group 2: frequency sweep 18 s, inverted, amplification 0.8 and frequency 1.15 kHz, inverted, amplification 18 fold

Fig. 34: Significant increase in the number of leucocytes and lymph nodes following bioresonance

Most **clinical trials** on bioresonance were conducted on **allergy patients**. This patient group is particularly suitable for trials as, in most cases, the effect of therapy is immediately perceptible to patients subjectively and can be observed by therapists. The disappearance of or improvement in a skin rash, a blocked nose, asthma or an intestinal complaint can easily be assessed.

Back in 1990 the paediatrician, Dr Schumacher, conducted a study in his practice of 204 children with various allergic conditions. The patients were interviewed and followed up between five and eleven months after the bioresonance therapy. 83% stated they no

What evidence is available?

longer had allergic symptoms. The symptoms had improved in 11% of respondents, only in 4.5% were they unchanged and 1.5% could not be assessed. At the time this was a revolutionary result, of which other forms of therapy could hardly dream. The level of evidence was rated 4-5.[28]

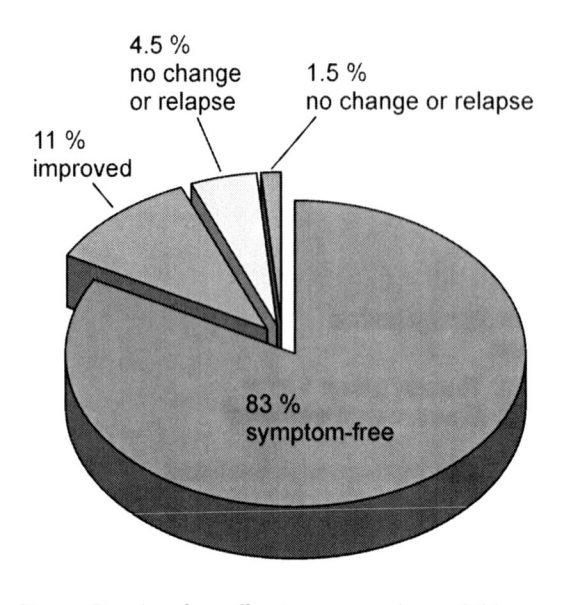

Fig. 35 Results of an effectiveness study on children with neurodermatitis (Dr. Schumacher).

During the same period Dr Schumacher published another study on **patients with hay fever**. The season following bioresonance therapy 43.4% experienced no symptoms while symptoms were improved in 50.4% of hay fever sufferers. This also represents a success rate of over 90%.[29]

In 1993 I conducted a study in my practice. Some months after developing and using meridian-related allergy therapy, I sent questionnaires to 248 patients who had mostly been treated with bioresonance but mostly without strict avoidance of the allergen concerned. The group included adults and children with **neurodermatitis, eczema, pollen allergy, allergic disorders of the eye, respiratory tract and intestines**. Of the 200 cases analysed, 50.4% stated they were symptom-free and 34.1% that their symptoms had improved. 15.5% reported no change. Most patients had a

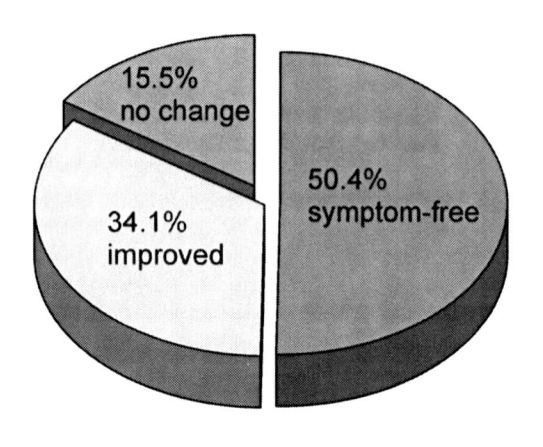

Fig. 36: Results of an allergy trial (Dr Hennecke).

---

[28] P. Schumacher: Ergebnisse der biophysikalischen Allergietherapie [Results of biophysical allergy therapy], in: Biophysikalische Therapie der Allergien [Biophysical allergy therapy], p. 125-129, Sonntag Verlag Stuttgart, 2004

[29] P. Schumacher: Biophysikalische Therapie des Heuschnupfens – Therapieergebnisse [Biophysical hayfever therapy-results], in: Biophysikalische Therapie der Allergien [Biophysical allergy therapy], S. 147-151, Sonntag Verlag, Stuttgart, 2004.

What evidence is available?

long history of allergy and had already undergone other less effective treatments.[30]

Between 2003 and 2006, a total of ten trials on allergy treatment were conducted in hospitals in the People's Republic of China and subsequently published. The results from, in some cases, large numbers of patients confirmed the positive results obtained from the practices. Most studies were carried out at the central hospital of the city of Xian, famous for the graves of the terracotta warriors.

An initial trial on 79 patients with **allergic skin disease** was published in March 2005. Here too, treatment resulted in almost 75% of patients being symptom-free and a further 22% experiencing an improvement in their symptoms.[31]

Efficacy rates of 60.8%[32] and 66.7% were also achieved in two trials on **chronic nettle rash**. A breakdown by age group in the first trial revealed the best results in the group aged between 1 and 15 (90%).[33]

Two trials dealt with **bronchial asthma** in children. In one study of 300 young asthmatics bioresonance therapy was compared to traditional asthma therapy with corticoids and anti-allergic agents.[34] As an expert assessor commented: "Conventional drug treatment is extremely effective, at least in treating symptoms. It is therefore astonishing that Bicom treatment achieves the same or even greater efficacy. The design has a high level of evidence: level 3 so that the results must be regarded as proof

---

[30] P. Schumacher: Biophysikalische Therapie des Heuschnupfens – Therapieergebnisse [Biophysical hay fever therapy - results], in: Biophysikalische Therapie der Allergien [Biophysical allergy therapy], p. 147-151, Sonntag Verlag, Stuttgart, 2004.

[31] Du Xia et al., Kinan Children's Hospital: Klinische Beobachtung über 79 Behandlungsfälle gegen allergische Hautkrankheiten mittels Bioresonanzgerät [Clinical observation of 79 cases of allergic skin disease treated with the bioresonance device], Chinese Journal of Practical Medicine, vol. 4, no. 3, 2005.

[32] Xu Minhong et al.: Klinische Beobachtung der Behandlung von chronischem Nesselausschlag mit dem Bioresonanzgerät [Clinical observation of treatment of chronic nettle rash with the bioresonance device], China Journal of Leprosy and Skin Diseases, vol. 21, no. 7, 2005

[33] Zhang X et al.: Klinische Beobachtung über 54 Behandlungsfälle gegen Nesselausschlag mittels BICOM Bioresonanzgerät [Clinical observation of 54 cases of nettle rash treated with the BICOM bioresonance device], Chinese Journal of Leprosy and Skin Disease, vol. 21, no. 8, 2005

[34] Yang Jinzhi and Zahn Li, research centre of Jinan Children's Hospital: 300 Behandlungsbeispiele gegen Asthma mittels BICOM Gerät bei Kinderpatienten [300 examples of treatment of asthma in children with the BICOM device], Maternal and Child Health Care of China, ISSN 1001-4411, 2004.

What evidence is available?

of efficacy."[35]

Another study compared three groups containing a total of 172 children with **bronchial asthma** or **allergic rhinitis**. The group which was treated purely with bioresonance did best (85.6% efficacy rate), closely followed by the group which was treated with the Bicom device after unsuccessful drug treatment (79.6%).

The worst result was recorded by the group solely receiving drug treatment (69.1% efficacy rate), evidence level 1-2.[36]

The largest study was a longitudinal observation of 1,639 patients (!) **with different allergic symptoms.**[37]

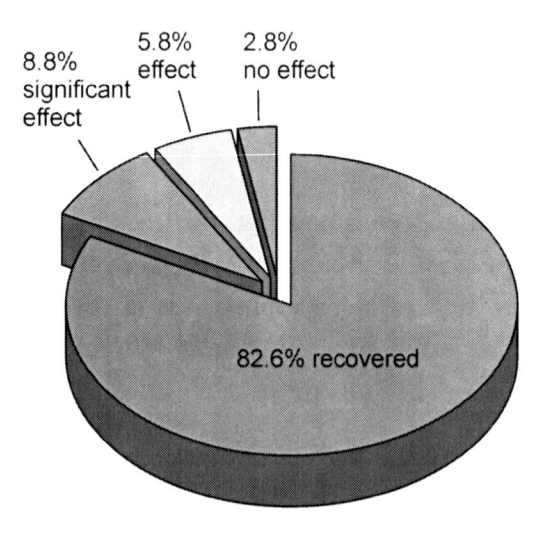

Pie chart: 82.6% recovered, 8.8% significant effect, 5.8% effect, 2.8% no effect.

Fig. 37: Paper presented at the 45th International Congress for BICOM Users: study of 1,639 asthma patients by Dr. med. Yuan Ze and Dr. med. Wang Haiyan, Xian Central Hospital.

Extract from the expert's assessment: The patients had previously been treated with various drugs with little success. The six-month symptom-free period following Bicom therapy indicates the patients were cured, for this period at least. Spontaneous healing, placebo effects or similar cannot explain the percentage of patients (83%) cured of these types of allergy. Level of evidence 4-5."[38]

One could get the impression that bioresonance is only suitable for treating allergies. In actual fact this method is used for a large number of different

---

[35] Data Analysis & Study Planning, Gauting: Expert opinion of 9.12.2005.

[36] Huan Shuiming et al.: Klinische Beobachtung der Behandlung von allergischem Schnupfen und Bronchialasthma von Kindern mit dem Bioresonanzgerät [Clinical observation of the treatment of allergic rhinitis and bronchial asthma in children with the bioresonance device], Zhe Jiang Medizinische Zeitschrift, edition 6, vol. 27, 2005.

[37] Yuan Ze and Wang Haiyan, Paediatric department of Xian Central Hospital: Klinische Ergebnisse mit dem BICOM 2000 Bioresonanzgerät [Clinical results with the BICOM 2000 bioresonance device], paper at the International Congress May 2005, Fulda, RTI-vol 29, Regumed Institut für Regulative Medizin.

[38] Data Analysis & Study Planning, Gauting: Expert opinion of 9.12.2005.

What evidence is available?

disorders. There are many reports of positive treatment and also some trials. These investigated damage to liver cells, functional intestinal complaints, sports injuries, arthroses and rheumatic disorders.

Laboratory values are extremely important in conventional medicine, both for diagnosis and for longitudinal observation of many disorders. They are considered scientifically objective since they are produced by a neutral laboratory device without the possible subjective influence of the therapist. They therefore receive particular attention in scientific work and have considerable evidentiary value. Can bioresonance exert a favourable influence on laboratory parameters or even bring them back to normal levels? Improved liver enzymes, renal functional values and thyroid parameters have repeatedly been observed in our practice. Individual cases are not sufficient evidence, however.

The result of a 1996 study of patients with **damage to their liver cells** is consequently all the more remarkable. A group of 14 patients in whom lab tests had detected liver damage was treated with bioresonance while a control group of 14 patients was left untreated. While the liver enzymes (gamma GT, GOT, GPT) of the control group remained virtually unchanged, these parameters improved significantly in the treated patients and even completely normalised in some. The study was rated evidence level 1 since it "leads to the conclusion that bioresonance has a high degree of statistically substantiated efficacy with this indication."[39]

Two other laboratory studies were conducted on patients with **rheumatoid arthritis**. Anti-oxidative enzymes in the lymphocytes (a subgroup of white blood corpuscles) were investigated. When rheumatism patients were treated purely with conventional medicine the activity levels of the enzymes peroxide dismutase, catalase and glutathione peroxidase were raised, while the thiol group content was lowered. Following additional bioresonance therapy, peroxide dismutase and glutathione peroxidase activity normalised, as did thiol group content. Although these findings may only be clear to specialists, an objective change in laboratory parameters is demonstrable with bioresonance. It may possibly activate non-specific protective mechanisms in patients with rheumatoid arthritis.[40]

---

[39] R. Machowinski and P. Kreisl: Prospektive randomisierte Studie zur Überprüfung der Behandlungserfolge mit patienteneigenen elektromag-netischen Feldern (BICOM) bei Leberfunktionsstörungen [Prospective randomised study to examine success of treatment of hepatic dysfunction with patients' own electromagnetic fields (BICOM)], in: Wissenschaftliche Studien [Scientific studies], Regumed Institut für Regulative Medizin, page 77-92, 1999.

[40] B. I. Islamov et al.: Effect of Bioresonance Therapy on Antioxidant System in Lymphocytes in Patients with Rheumatoid Arthritis, Bulletin of Experimental Biology and Medicine, no. 3, 248-250, 2002.

What evidence is available?

Another study investigated heat shock protein synthesis which is reduced to 60% in patients with rheumatoid arthritis. These values returned to normal under the influence of bioresonance. The author assumes that the observed therapeutic effect of bioresonance in rheumatism patients is connected with an improvement in lymphocyte activity, brought about by normalisation of heat shock protein synthesis.[41]

But there are also clinical studies on muscle and joint problems. Two patient groups with fibromyalgia syndrome were treated with physiotherapy and point massage. One group was also given bioresonance therapy. Both groups stated their condition had improved. However, the effect was felt more frequently and sooner in the bioresonance group and was also stronger and more prolonged than in the control group. Muscular pain (muscular syndrome index) improved by 72% with bioresonance (37% for control group). Sleeping disorders and sensitivity to changes in the weather also improved significantly compared with the control group.[42]

While functional muscular and joint pain tends to play a part in fibromyalgia, the symptoms of arthrosis are usually caused by signs of wear in the joints and associated inflammatory changes. Can bioresonance offer help and support here too?

A study of patients with **arthrosis of the knee joint (gonarthrosis)** produced sensational results. Two patient groups received conventional medical treatment. One group was also treated with bioresonance. The pain symptoms eased much quicker in the bioresonance group and were checked by the therapy for a much longer period. The success of the treatment was judged by criteria such as joint pain, joint function, blood analysis, well-being and fitness for work. Accordingly a success rate of 94% was recorded in the bioresonance group, with the control group scoring 57.5%. Joint sonography alone revealed a 75% improvement following bioresonance treatment compared with 32.5% for the control group.[43]

The joints of top athletes are subject to an extreme degree of strain and there is consider-

---

[41] B. I. Islamov et al.: Bioresonance Therapy of Rheumatoid Arthritis and Heat Shock Proteins, Bulletin of Experimental Biology and Medicine, no. 11, 1112-1115, 1999.

[42] F. F. Gogoleva: New Approaches to Diagnosis and Treatment of Fibromyalgia in Spinal Osteochondrosis, Ter Arkh., 73(4), 40-5, 2002.

[43] Maiko Olu, Gogoleva F. F.: Outpatient Bioresonance Treatment of Gonarthrosis, Ter Arkh, 2002, 72(12), 50-3.

What evidence is available?

able risk of injury. Some sports associations and even Olympic teams are already exploiting the therapeutic benefits of bioresonance. In a study a group of twelve top athletes with excessive strain was treated purely with bioresonance, while a second group of twelve sportsmen was treated purely with conventional methods such as ultrasonics, stimulation current, cryotherapy and anti-rheumatic agents. While the efficacy was the same, the therapy time was shorter for the bioresonance group and fewer treatment sessions were required.[44]

Another study revealed a positive effect in patients with **functional gastrointestinal problems**. The symptoms improved by 48.2% in the bioresonance group and by only 3.8% in the placebo group.[45]

The opponents of the bioresonance method have not been resting on their laurels naturally. At any rate, there have been two(!) studies which apparently showed that bioresonance was ineffective. A study on **hay fever** patients was printed in a specialist journal in 1996. The therapy was not conducted in line with usual correct procedures, however.

Contrary to recommendations in the literature and in the training seminars, testing and treatment was conducted with skin prick solutions. It was also already known at that time that unmodified allergens are far more likely to prove successful for therapy. The result was interesting despite bioresonance therapy not being conducted in ideal onditions. 5 of the 42 patients in the bioresonance group nevertheless indicated they were symptom-free and 18 had seen their symptoms improve (a success rate of over 50%). Only two (25%) of the eight patients in the placebo group reported an improvement. The result is not statistically relevant due to the low number of patients. In conclusion the author claimed that this study provided proof that bioresonance does **not** work.[46]

---

[44] B. J. Pape_, Joze Barovic, Maribor Teaching Hospital, Medical Rehabilitation Dept.. led by Chief physician Zmago Turk: Bericht über die Verwendung der BICOM Resonanz-Therapie beim Überlastungs-Syndrom von Hochleistungs- sportlern [Report on the use of BICOM resonance therapy for excessive strain in top athletes] ; Wissenschaftliche Studien [Scientific studies], Regumed Institut für Regulative Medizin, 1999.

[45] J. Niehaus, M. Galle: Placebokontrollierte Studie zur Wirkung einer standardisierten Mora-Bioresonanz-Therapie auf funktionelle Magen-Darm-Beschwerden [Placebo-controlled study on the effect of standardised Mora bioresonance therapy on functional gastrointestinal complaints], Forschende Komplementärmedizin, 13, p. 28-34, 2006.

[46] H. Kofler et al.: Department of Dermatology, University Innsbruck: Bioresonance in diagnosis and treatment of hay fever; unpublished.

What evidence is available?

What is even more astonishing is that allergologists, specialists and experts kept quoting this study at conferences and in the press and playing it up to disprove bioresonance therapy.

Another counter study was carried out in 1997 in the well-known children's hospital in Davos. 32 children with **neurodermatitis** were treated in accordance with conventional medical guidelines with cortisone, antibiotics, urea and crystal violet. Half of the patients also received bioresonance therapy. Unfortunately the guidelines recommended in training were not followed correctly in this case either. In the end no difference was detected between the results for the two groups. It was concluded from this that bioresonance has no effect.[47] Word has got around, even amongst non-medical professionals, that cortisone gets rid of virtually every case of neurodermatitis symptoms (temporarily). Consequently additional treatment cannot improve the situation further! Naturally it's not possible to prove anything with a study design like that.

To my knowledge no further counter studies have appeared in the literature since these two works. Nevertheless, publications are repeatedly issued by scientists and journalists which, either from ignorance or deliberately, disregard the current state of research and claim that "bioresonance is not scientifically proven." The lack of objective arguments in these publications is often replaced by polemic.

This is not a new phenomenon. No less a personage than Johann Wolfgang von Goethe noted in a discussion on professors who still present outdated theories although these have long since been refuted by new research work: "They do not prove the truth and that is not their intention at all. They are merely concerned with proving their opinion. Consequently they also hide all the experiments which would bring the truth to light and expose the untruthfulness of their teaching."

Bioresonance therapy works. The studies described above prove this. But what is the situation as regards **energetic diagnosis** which is mainly used as the basis for therapy? A number of studies have also been conducted on this subject. **Voll's electroacupuncture (EAV)**, in particular, has been compared with traditional methods. An American study

---

[47] M. Schöni et al.: Efficacy Trial of Bioresonance in Children with Atopic Dermatitis, Int. Arch Allergy-Immunology, 112-238-246, 1997.

What evidence is available?

back in 1984 revealed a high degree of agreement between EAV testing and conventional diagnosis.[48]

In a 2002 Italian study the results of EAV testing were compared with the prick test on 31 patients with four allergies (mites, grasses, olive tree, pellitory of the wall). The level of agreement was 95%. When evaluating this study it was observed that, "as an objective method, the Bicom device is highly suited to conducting allergy tests." This study was rated evidence level 1.[49] Two further studies from China confirmed these positive results.[50]

In a 2001 randomised double blind trial no correlation between EAV and the prick test was found.[51] What produced this contrary result? Did the quality of the test series or the quality of the tester play a crucial role here?

Tensor testing also appears to have failed in a 1993 comparative study.[52] The investigations took place on blood samples during a laboratory inspection and definitely cannot be assessed by the criteria of scientific studies.

In actual fact we also repeatedly experience differences in our own practice between conventional medical results brought in by patients and our own energetic testing.

The results of prick tests depend on the test serum used and on the analyst's interpretation. Otherwise there would be no explanation why patients who consult several allergy specialists sometimes bring widely differing test results with them. The prick test

---

[48] Julia J. Tsuei et al.: A Food Allergy Study Utilizing the EAV Acupuncture Technique, American Journal of Acupuncture, vol. 12, no. 2, 105-116, 1984.

[49] E. Giannazz et al., Catania University: Diagnosi Allergologiche con Tecnologie Biofisiche; Catania Medica, 9-11, 2002.

[50] Liu Xiaoku: Anwendung der Bioresonanz-Technik bei allergischen Krankheiten – Analyse der häufigsten Allergien in der Stadt Xiamen [Use of the bioresonance method with allergic disorders – analysis of the most common allergies in Xiamen], Chinese Journal of Leprosy and Skin Disease, vol. 21, no. 9, 2005; and Yang Xiaoying, Liu Qiang, Shanxi Province Children's Hospital: Untersuchung der Bioresonanztechnik zur Prüfung atopischer Dermatitis [Investigation of the bioresonance technique for testing atopic dermatitis], Shanxi Medical Journal, ISSN 0253-9926, 2005.

[51] George T. Lewith et al.: Is electrodermal testing as effective as skin prick tests for diagnosing allergies, A double blind, randomised block design study; BMJ, Volume 322, 121-134, 2001.

[52] F. Wantke et al.: Bioresonanz-Allergietest versus Pricktest und Rast, Kurze wissenschaftliche Mitteilung [Bioresonance allergy test versus prick test and RAST, a short scientific report], Allergologie, year 16, no. 4, 144-145, 1993.

indicates sensitisation. Sensitisation is not the same as an apparent allergy.[53]

It is only classed as an allergy if appropriate symptoms are also present. They can be confirmed by a provocation test if necessary. Unfortunately patients are often misinformed here too. Many people display sensitisation to house dust mites in the prick test yet only patients with a clinically apparent allergy react to them with a running nose or shortness of breath.

According to experience in my practice, energetic test methods indicate much better what substances patients actually react to. Patients very often confirm the test result based on their own observations. It is of no significance here whether this is a genuine atopic allergy, a pseudoallergy or an intolerance. This is not important for therapy with bioresonance.

While we often find agreement with the prick test in the case of inhalational allergies (mites, mould, pollen, animal hair), the results often differ significantly when it comes to food allergies. Even the results of different conventional medical skin and antibody tests rarely concur. Senior allergy specialists believe there are no conventional medical or alternative test methods which can prove a food allergy with a sufficiently high degree of certainty. Only an oral provocation test after avoiding the food in question for a prolonged period can provide definite proof.[54] This potentially worthwhile but very laborious method is not really feasible in daily practice..

In the case of food allergies and intolerance, a well trained and experienced tester can diagnose the right offending substances with a high degree of probability. If the condition improves following bioresonance therapy applied on this basis, this proves the diagnosis was correct.

---

[53] Sensibilisierung ist keine Allergie [Sensitisation is not an allergy], Medical Tribune no. 42, 20.10.2006.

[54] Tebbe, Lepp, Niggemann, Werfel: „Nahrungsmittelallergie und -Unverträglichkeit: Bewährte statt nicht evaluierte Diagnostik" [Food allergy and intolerance. Proven rather than unevaluated diagnosis], Deutsches Ärzteblatt 102, vol 27, 1965 – 1969, 2005.

What evidence is available?

Numerous studies are now available which have been conducted in line with scientific criteria and which conclusively prove the effect of the bioresonance method. These include in-vitro studies and clinical trials, in some cases with a high evidence level (1–2). Clinical trials with large numbers of patients and a conclusive positive result have been carried out in China.

Frequently asked questions

Why doesn't conventional medicine recognise bioresonance?

Lets us take the example of allergies. They represent a challenge and the opportunities for treating them with conventional medicine are often highly unsatisfactory. If there was just the slightest suspicion that new therapeutic approaches could bring relief, ethically oriented research should jump upon them with scientific enthusiasm. It would take very little time to determine whether the new method was a waste of time or whether something genuinely valuable lay behind it. For, ultimately, allergies are a condition which affects millions of people and responsibility for the nation's health is at stake. And why isn't this the case?

Who are the authorities in Germany who determine what is scientifically recognised or not? The universities and the courts! Universities are traditionally the centres of modern scientific research. Research is costly and becoming ever more so. The funding universities receive from the state for research work has been inadequate for some time. Consequently sponsors are needed. Research work is commissioned and paid for by the pharmaceutical industry and other sectors of industry. University professors responsible for the research can also boost their salaries by this means. It is quite natural to wonder how objective and neutral research actually is today. You would also expect that careful study design would always produce the same or similar results. Far from the truth. How often do we read studies of the same topic with totally different, even contradictory results! There is little interest in alternative methods which are not backed by big investors. Professors who tackle these subjects have to fear for their jobs in certain circumstances.

As experts in their field, university professors are the highest authority for legal opinions. In case of doubt the judges decide, based on these opinions, what is the scientifically accepted standard (and thus that accepted by conventional medicine) and what isn't.

There are plenty of examples from the past of how 'official' conventional medicine has long held up progress. Just think of the recommended hygiene procedures to prevent childbed fever and the discovery of penicillin. Ultimately the right methods have gained acceptance in the end. But it takes time. As the physicist Max Planck said: "Not only the

Frequently asked questions

professors, but their students, need to die out for a new scientific idea to gain acceptance." But we no longer have this much time today.

The pressure for new developments now no longer comes from above (science and politics) but from below (general public). The studies to recognise acupuncture were not proposed by the universities. The pressure from patients and therapists became so great that it was no longer possible to avoid tackling the subject. But it took nearly forty years.

So it is not surprising if a relatively new method (although it has already been in existence over 30 years) is not exactly welcomed with open arms, especially if it means the scientific world view will have to be corrected (once more).

Traditionally people initially fight against every new idea since they don't want to move away from the long-standing structures. If that no longer works, they simply ignore the method including all the success stories and studies associated with it. Sometimes it is the opponents who involuntarily help a method gain recognition. An 'admonition association' instituted legal proceedings so that, like it or not, the courts had to tackle the subject of bioresonance.

Following a five-year legal battle and based on the situation as regards clinical trials, the Munich higher regional court has now officially allowed the claim "the bioresonance method can diagnose and effectively treat allergies" to be used in advertising.

Why won't health insurance funds cover bioresonance?

Let's just pose a counter question: what would happen if a large number of all the doctors in practices and hospitals treated most of their patients with bioresonance? Many patients would possibly get better quicker with fewer side effects and less cost for the health system. Far less medication and other medical procedures would be required. There are definitely interest groups who would object to this. This would threaten jobs and the entire health policy would need rethinking. Can we ask this of our politicians? The health insurance funds are not really the restricting factor in this.

In the mid-1990s virtually all the health insurance funds paid part of the cost of bioresonance therapy, especially if it helped and rendered other procedures unnecessary. Some funds even sent us patients, for example children with neurodermatitis, because they saw the positive results.

As part of the various health reforms a commission was set up which decides which treatment methods may be reimbursed by the health insurance funds. Who sits on this commission? Along with numerous other alternative methods bioresonance was dropped from the list! The health insurance funds are no longer allowed to reimburse bioresonance, even if they wanted to! Instead of explaining this political decision honestly to patients, when asked health insurance fund employees repeatedly claim that bioresonance is not reimbursed because it does not work.

Why do we hear so little about bioresonance in the media?

Television, radio stations and newspapers are unfortunately not as politically independent as we would wish. What the public can and cannot be informed about is seemingly subject to selection. The opinion of (selected) experts is then intended to influence the shaping of public opinion.

In the past there were repeatedly broadcasts or newspaper articles about bioresonance. Some of these were totally dismissive, while others allowed people with positive experiences to have their say. Apparently a probably unintentional consequence of this was that even negative reports arouse the interest of the public. Along the lines of, if there is so much opposition to a method, then there must be something in it! Then all the reports on bioresonance appeared to stop at once. Instead all the glossy magazines carry reports at regular intervals about the ways of treating allergies with conventional medicine. One cannot help feeling that these articles have been copied time and again with slight differences for 30 years.

Why does nobody report on the clinical trials for bioresonance or on the verdict of the Munich higher regional court? That would be really sensational! But people won't let themselves be taken for idiots. Today everyone is able to find out about all kinds of subjects through the internet. Here you can find negative and positive reports on bioresonance. Everyone can form their own opinion. The influence of the media is often overestimated anyway. Most patients don't go to therapists' practices as a result of reports

Frequently asked questions

in the media but because of word-of-mouth, in other words, on the recommendation of other patients who have been helped by this method. And patients treated successfully then recommend it in turn. This development can no longer be stopped.

What side-effects are observed with bioresonance?

Bioresonance is a regulatory method of treatment, similar to homeopathy, acupuncture and physiotherapy. A medication triggers biochemical processes in the body at the material level. The effects on the various organs are mostly well-known and reproducible biochemically. It is possible to clearly distinguish between the desired (therapeutic) effects and the adverse (side-)effects.

With methods of regulatory therapy such as bioresonance, the body is given an impulse to which it should react. The right impulse triggers a chain of biochemical reactions in the body which activate the organism's powers of self healing to take countermeasures against the causes of the disorder. An incorrect impulse has no or minimal effect. Consequently, if using the bioresonance method properly, it is difficult to do something completely wrong.

Side-effects in the conventional medical sense have not so far been observed by bioresonance therapists. Adverse reactions following therapy may be initial exacerbation or primary immune responses. They are encountered in all methods of regulatory therapy.

An initial exacerbation is generally a sign that the therapy impulse was definitely the right one but the strength of the impulse was too intensive. This leads to a temporary worsening of the symptoms, intensification of the pain or of the skin eczema, for example. It can also happen that old symptoms from the past, from which the patient had apparently recovered, reappear. Sometimes teeth, which were chronically inflamed yet previously displayed no symptoms, also make their presence felt. If old foci flare up, this can give therapists important clues about hidden therapy blocks.

Reactions such as this in which the patient's condition deteriorates usually subside within one or two days yet may last longer in individual cases. At the next treatment session the therapist will adapt the therapy according to the individual patient's responsiveness.

Frequently asked questions

Constant over-treatment can, in the worst case, lead to reaction blocks. But even these can generally be overcome with treatment to restore the energy balance.

It is not unusual therefore for the symptoms of chronic disorders not to improve continuously but rather for the patient's condition to fluctuate somewhat at the start of the treatment. The therapist and patient may need to be patient at this stage.

Patients with autoimmune disorders should be treated with care as they often have a tendency to hyperintensive reactions. Patients should not be given bioresonance therapy during the first three months of pregnancy for forensic reasons.

If therapy fails to be successful, although not a side-effect, this can be problematical in certain cases. If a patient who is known to have violent reactions, e.g. asthma attacks or shock reactions, is treated for allergy, any exposure test should only be conducted under clinical conditions. No test, neither conventional medical nor energetic allergy test, can predict with one hundred percent certainty whether exposure to the allergen will cause a reaction in the patient or not. Emergency medication should continue to be carried as a precaution.

Does bioresonance therapy help everyone and with all disorders?

There is no medical method in the world which will help everyone. Man is not a machine which runs according to technically reproducible rules. Every person is an individual and disease should be regarded as a largely multifactorial product of physical, psychological and social circumstances. Organs and tissue which are completely destroyed or missing cannot be restored by any method, not even bioresonance. Deficient enzymes, vitamins and nutrients must also be physically supplied. Applying a food's biophysical information to a patient will not satiate their hunger! Provided responsive tissue is still present, an improvement can often be brought about in the patient's condition through bioresonance. Oscillation patterns which are superior to matter will often produce an effect where chemical substances are no longer effective at the physical level.

Severe psychological trauma cannot be treated with bioresonance either. A difficult childhood, abuse, traumatic events and chronic frustration can cause or encourage illness or impede its treatment. The bioresonance device cannot change mothers-in-law or partners! There are also patients who derive benefit from their illness, usually subconsciously. While they are ill, they are guaranteed the affection and care of their partner and family. Or they have a reason not to have to go to work. There are patients who run from one therapist to another and try everything to continually receive confirmation that they are incurably ill. When they feel that they are getting better, the therapy is discontinued with often flimsy excuses. Patients who have applied for sickness-related benefits are often untreatable.

You have perhaps noticed in reading this that I have never used the word 'cure'. Bioresonance can relieve the symptoms of many medical conditions or even make them disappear. Whether the patient is completely cured depends largely upon his mental attitude to the disorder and upon other psychological and social factors. Many therapists combine the bioresonance method with other conventional medical and naturopathic methods of therapy. A sensitive therapeutic discussion can often work wonders!

Experienced bioresonance therapists report an 80-90% success rate, depending on the patient group. One patient in nine or ten unfortunately cannot be helped. Every, otherwise good, practice has its share of failures. All therapists must learn to deal with this. For we aren't 'gods in white coats'. We should learn to accept failure and concentrate on the success stories. The 80:20 rule is well known in economics. We spend 20% of our working time on 80% of our (routine) patients and 80% of our time on 20% of our (difficult) patients.

The reason for therapy failing may be an undiscovered or untreated physical or psychological therapy block. Or perhaps the right allergen or toxin or responsible germ hasn't been found? Or it may be that the therapist is not sufficiently experienced. We should not be afraid of referring a patient to another therapist. Patents and therapists not only enter into a treatment contract enshrined in law. The chemistry, or as we would now more accurately say, the vibes must be right. Interpersonal dissonance is not a good basis for therapy. To sum up, bioresonance is a method of diagnosing and treating patients which provides relief to very many disorders and can help cure the patient.

Concluding remarks

We are now witnessing the end of an era where medical conditions are treated using solely drug-based biochemical means. The information age has already begun and is having a profound impact on medical science too. In the future techniques that embrace biophysical information transfer will become the norm. The bioresonance method represents an important milestone on this journey.

Glossary

Acupuncture point: Point defined in Traditional Chinese Medicine on the surface of the body, generally on a meridian pathway, used for energetic diagnosis or therapy.

Output cup: A cup-shaped electrode for holding information carriers, usually in liquid form, for example, special mineral solutions or energetically processed and natural sesame oil, in order to apply therapeutic information to them (individualise).

Bandpass: A narrow frequency range within a larger frequency range which passes through a filter for certain therapy functions. The frequency ranges above and below are suppressed.

Cup electrode: A cup-shaped electrode used both for the device input and output. The cup electrode for the device input is used to hold substances to enable their energetic information to flow into the therapeutic control circuit. The cup electrode for the device output is used to hold information carriers, for example, special mineral solutions or energetically processed and natural sesame oil, in order to apply therapeutic information to them.

Biophoton: Photons or light waves which a cell, a cell group or living organism emits or absorbs. They act as information carriers.

Bioresonance: The capacity of a biological system to react to waves and frequency patterns by resonating. In the narrower sense, a form of therapy in which an organism is encouraged by its body's natural frequency pattern or that of a substance to respond by self-regulating.

Bioresonance method: A method of diagnosing and treating with the body's natural frequency patterns and those of substances.

Chip storage device: A device with which stainless steel chips are loaded with therapeutic frequency information. They are placed on the body to prolong and intensify therapy.

Chirality: Mirror-image arrangement of structures, for example, biochemical molecules,

Glossary

with otherwise identical design.

Sweeping bandpass: A narrow frequency range which runs through the entire frequency range available within a specified period (in seconds).

Input cup: A cup-shaped electrode for holding substances to enable their energetic information to flow into the therapeutic control circuit.

Flexible electrode: Contact electrode made of flexible material which adapts to the shape of the area of the body.

Frequency sweep: A narrow frequency range which runs through the entire frequency range available within a predetermined period.

Frequency pattern: Oscillations of specific frequencies which are emitted by all organic and non-organic substances, including the body's cells. Due to their wave properties they form different patterns which are also used to transmit information.

Five element theory: Part of Traditional Chinese Medicine, for explaining the energy flow in the body and in the meridians. The five elements (feedback circuits) are designated the names fire, water, wood, metal and earth. Each element is made up of two or four classic acupuncture meridians. The classic idea was extended in Voll's electroacupuncture.

Basic therapy: BICOM therapy is generally initiated with basic therapy, designed to prepare the body for the actual specific therapy.

Background contamination/basic stress: Pathological exacerbating factors such as bacteria, viruses, toxic substances, chronic allergies which often manifest themselves in the body in early years and are partly responsible for causing or sustaining a medical condition. Therapy may prove unsuccessful if these are not identified.

Information transfer: The oscillations with specific frequency patterns which are emitted by the body's cells or other substances also contain information. They can be transmitted to other substances or parts of the body by means of an appropriate therapy device.

Glossary

Infrared transmitter: An auxiliary device which feeds the frequency pattern of a substance into the therapy device by means of infrared beams and does not require a cable connection. It is used in energetic testing to determine from a relatively large number of ampoules or preparations in as rational a manner as possible what is affecting the body.

Inverting: Shifting the phase of a wave electronically by 180°, making minus plus and vice versa.

Kinesiology: Study of movement: Technique for testing and restoring the energy balance of impaired muscle function. The muscle test is used in connection with the bioresonance method to diagnose pathological influences based on energy flow and to determine appropriate therapy programs and medication.

Focus of disease: A local accumulation of pathogens and toxins resulting from a medical condition from which the patient did not completely recover and which can affect more distant areas of the body.

Magnet electrode: Electrode with a relatively strong magnetic field to transfer the therapeutic information into even deeper-lying areas of the body.

Medication test: Part of an energetic test procedure, for example electroacupuncture, with whose help the medication or implant which is appropriate or effective for the patient can be identified.

Meridian: Energy pathways determined according to Traditional Chinese Medicine and running over the surface of the body which connect acupuncture points.

Meridian flooding: A form of therapy used in connection with bioresonance therapy whereby an acupuncture meridian can be energetically stimulated or suppressed.

Meridian point: See acupuncture point.

Meridian therapy: See meridian flooding.

Measured value: In electroacupuncture testing the energetic state of an acupuncture

Glossary

point and that of the organ area assigned to it is indicated on a scale of 10 to 100 units. A distinction is made, in terms of energy, between a chronic degenerative state, a normal state and an acute inflammatory state.

Centre frequency: The middle frequency of a defined band pass.

Modulation mat: A special output electrode with a pancake coil which produces an extremely weak magnetic field. This field has a substantial depth effect in the body however.

Pathological frequency pattern: In the healthy state, the cells of an organ area have a specific frequency spectrum with which they communicate with one another. If a pathogen or a toxic substance penetrates a cell or even the intercellular space, the frequency spectrum in this area changes. Pathological frequency patterns arise which can develop a clinical picture if the body is no longer able to compensate for them. All disorders correlate with pathological frequency patterns.

Ability to regulate: The ability of the body to maintain or restore its physiological and energetic balance in the face of pathogenic influences.

Resonance phenomena: All physical bodies, both inanimate and animate, have complex frequency patterns with specific functions and information which are able to resonate with other (e.g. electromagnetic) oscillations.

Oscillatory information: The frequency patterns originating from the body or from an external source of radiation are capable of exchanging and storing information.

Radiation exposure: The human body is subjected to a multitude of natural or technically generated radiation fields (e.g. radio waves, radar, computers) which severely impair the body's natural regulation and can lead to regulatory disorders or to illness.

Therapy type: In BICOM therapy the body's natural oscillations or frequency patterns are selected and combined into six different types to encourage the body to self regulate and eliminate the pathological state.

Glossary

Therapy block: Influences manifest in the body which impede the flow of energy in the body and thus the progress of therapy.

Therapy program: Combination of oscillation parameters such as type of therapy, amplification (amplitude), bandpass, therapy time, etc. to provide electronically pre-set therapy guidelines (empirical).

Amplification sweep: The amplification of a frequency pattern (amplitude) is continuously raised starting from the lowest level or lowered from the highest to the lowest level.

Wobbling bandpass: A narrow bandpass which moves back and forth within a limited range and can therefore reach a greater frequency range with simultaneous phase shift.

Honeycomb (test honeycomb): An electrode with several separate compartments for holding several test ampoules at once.

Photo credits

Photos and diagrams Jürgen Hennecke, apart from:

Figure 1 Medizinische Literarische Verlagsgesellschaft mbH, Uelzen
Figure 2 Med-Tronik GmbH, Friesenheim
Figure 4, 6, 7, 9, 11, 21, 22 Regumed GmbH, Gräfelfing
Figure 10 and 17 Jürgen Hennecke, Allergie und Schwingung, Astro-Spiegel-Verlag
Figure 19 and 20 Martha Schütte, Linz
Figure 15, 16, 23, 24, 25, 29, 30 Ulrich Wirth, Düsseldorf
Figure 26, 27, 28 Sabine Buller, Roetgen
Figure 32 Digital Stock